c b
c o°

Clean Beauty

Recipes to manage your beauty routine, *naturally*

By Elsie Rutterford
and Dominika
Minarovic,
Clean Beauty Co.

SQUARE PEG, LONDON

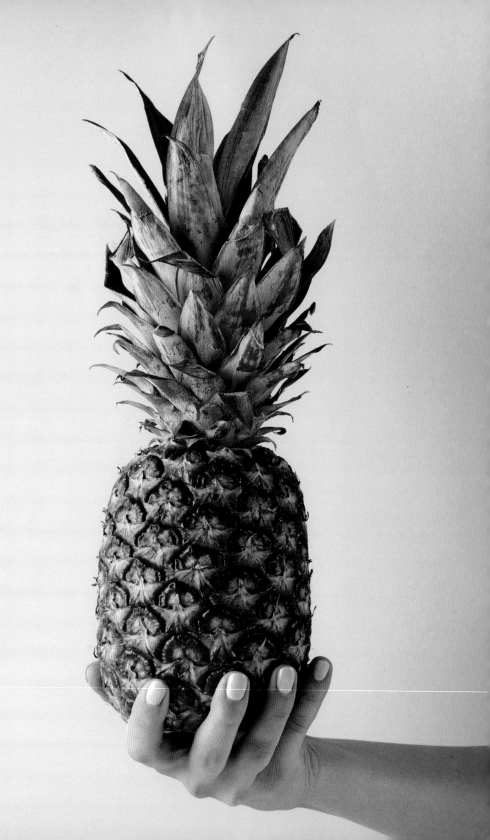

CONTENTS

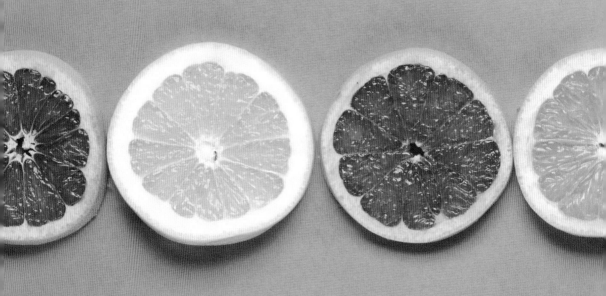

coming clean

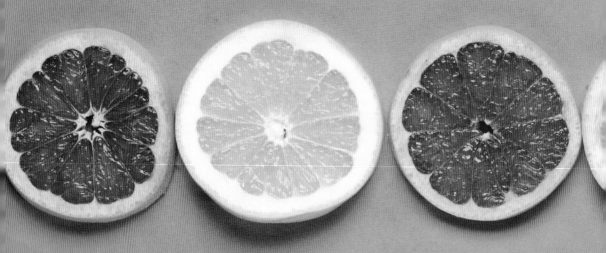

what is this clean beauty lark?

We all know we should read our food labels these days, turning our noses up at additives, strange E numbers and added sugars. We're so used to chucking the contents of our veg drawer (green or otherwise) into the NutriBullet and sipping it from our biodegradable, reusable canisters on the way to Bikram. We all get that health, fitness and well-being are intrinsically linked and we're all doing our best to change our lifestyles for the better. And that's great, we're totally on board. But in the flurry of whipping up another batch of vegan protein balls, many of us are overlooking another daily routine that has become pretty much second nature since our teenage years: one that's just as important to our health and well-being.

So we're turning our attention to our beauty products and applying the same thought process: if I care about what I put *in* my body, what about what I slather *all over it*? Clean beauty means using products that contain high quantities of natural ingredients and are totally clear of any questionable ingredients that don't benefit our bodies in any way. Clean beauty is about using our beauty routine to nourish our skin and hair, just as we use food to nourish and fuel our bodies. The cleaner and simpler we keep our products, the healthier we can be. The body absorbs what is put onto it, so seeking out unprocessed, nutrient-rich ingredients makes sense. We're not wasting our money on cheap alternatives; we're actually feeding our skin and hair with high quantities of our favourite plants, nuts, flowers and seeds: all the anti-ageing, super-moisturising, ultra-nourishing goodness that hasn't been diluted with pointless fillers.

What's more, we're all aware that our planet is deteriorating. Clean beauty is also about sustainability: ethical manufacturing processes, eco-friendly packaging; using less and wasting less; all helping to protect our environment.

We love beauty products but we also love our health. And this is what clean beauty means to us: absolute potency, zero fillers, 100 per cent natural. Want to know more? Join the movement #cleanbeautycrew.

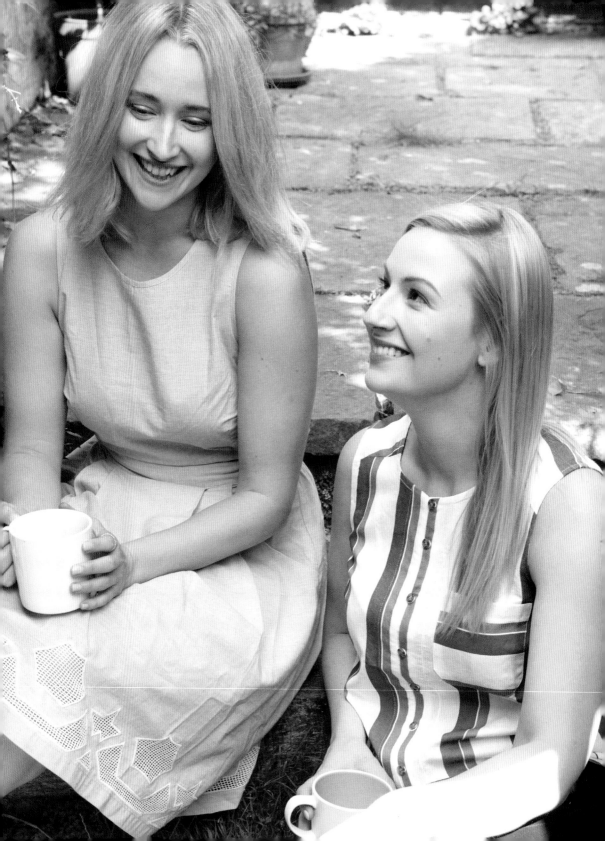

our story

We're Dominika and Elsie, founders of Clean Beauty Co. We met in advertising in 2013 when we both joined the same media company. It wasn't long before we became firm work BFFs: bonding over office gossip and online shopping. Our real common ground was a shared passion for health and well-being. We were regular gym buddies, spurring each other on to do that extra set of squats or one more press-up. We embarked on some physically testing (and downright crazy) challenges together, including a 64-mile walk to Brighton (never again) and an Olympic-distance triathlon. We also embraced the healthy eating trends that had taken the UK by storm, exploring new ways of eating. Vegan, Paleo, Lean in 15 ... You name it we tried it and we loved exploring what fuels our bodies. We were scrutinising food labels, growing savvy to unnecessary added sugars and additives and shifting our diets away from processed foods.

Alongside this we were also, like many twenty-somethings living in London, complete beauty fanatics. Working in sales meant we were expected to regularly entertain clients and we loved nothing more than a trip to the spa with them (tough gig). Manicures, pedicures, facials, waxing, tinting, dyeing and general pruning and preening; we were (and still are) absolute beauty junkies and were willing at that time to pay anything for the latest miracle cream.

It was a combination of these two – our love for both health and beauty – that ignited an idea. We were passionate about what was going *into* our bodies ... but had we stopped to think what was going *onto* our bodies? Had we ever actually read the labels of our moisturisers, creams, scrubs, soaks, hair oils, body washes, shampoos and conditioners?

Despite an overwhelming urge to turn a blind eye, we decided to brave up and take a quick peek at the ingredients list of one of our beloved products. Needless to say, when we looked we were both disappointed and pretty shocked. What were these long lists of ingredients that we couldn't even pronounce? Were they really the healthy, age-defying, ultra-nourishing power ingredients that the industry promises? In short, no. Of course they weren't. There were synthetic fillers, pointless additions, water: all there to make more of a product at a much cheaper price. And on even closer inspection, there were some pretty alarming ingredients lurking in our favourite products. After a little research, we realised that the stuff we were slathering all over our faces, on our mouths and close to our eyes – and paying all that money for the privilege – could be potentially hazardous to our health. Ouch. It was enough of a shock to kick us into taking action. We decided to make a change and, pretty much overnight, Clean Beauty Co. was born.

At that point we were faced with a decision — we could go on a shopping spree and replace every product on our bathroom shelves with natural alternatives, which would be an easy thing to do. There are some amazing brands out there making effective, clean beauty products. But we wanted to take things a step further, to pull apart our products, understand exactly what was going into them and try to replicate this process ourselves. We were doing the same with food, after all — making fresh, unprocessed and wholefood recipes inspired by the likes of Deliciously Ella, Madeleine Shaw and the Hemsley sisters. So surely we could do the same with our beauty products?

Turns out we were right. Making our own beauty products is totally doable and actually much easier, more enjoyable and, most importantly, more effective than we thought. We're in complete control over every single ingredient that we put all over our bodies, and our skin and hair has never looked better. Our company (and this book) is the result of hours of study, practice and a diploma in Natural Skincare Formulation. We're experts now and we want to share everything we've learnt. We've done the hard work for you, bringing you a curated collection of our very best natural DIY beauty recipes that really work, and won't harm your skin or the planet in the process.

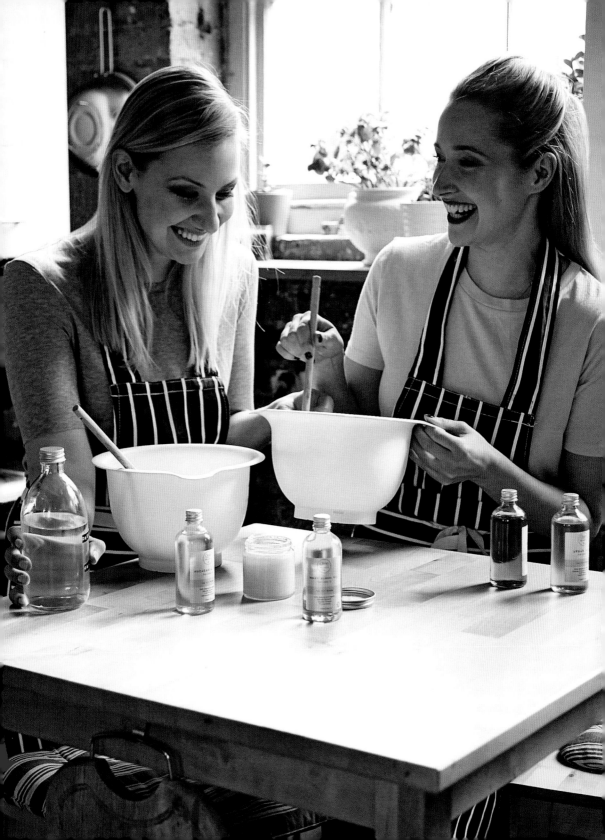

getting started

What you need, apart from all the ingredients, obvs:

• Mixing bowls

• Digital kitchen scales that measure down to 0.1 grams

• A pot and glass bowl for a bain-marie

• Aluminium spoons (wood harbours bacteria faster and other types of metal shouldn't be used with ingredients such as clay. Invest in a good set of aluminium spoons and you can use them for all of your recipes)

• Plastic funnels

• 50ml glass jars

• 120ml glass jars

• 50ml glass bottles with atomiser cap (amber bottles are best if you can find them)

• 50ml glass bottles with pump cap (ditto)

• Ice cube and muffin trays

• Hairnets

• Disposable gloves

• An apron

So now you know what kit you need (not much, right?). We know you're probably eager to throw yourself headfirst into the kitchen and begin concocting a fabulous range of non-toxic, luxurious and nutrition-packed goodies to grace your bathroom shelf. But just hold up a couple of minutes, would you? We hate to be party poopers but there are a couple of things we absolutely have to run through before we let you loose. It may seem tedious but the information over the next few pages is incredibly important and if it is not read and followed thoroughly, you run the risk of putting your health and safety at risk, which sort of defeats the object, doesn't it?

measurements

We've tried to make these recipes feel accessible, so your first step into DIY beauty isn't a daunting one. We've translated our formulas into babe-friendly language; you'll notice half a mashed banana here and a full cup there. Rest assured, these are all tried and tested recipes and we've made sure the measurements translate. And the scientific brains among you will note we're using a mix of ml, g and drops. Traditional formulas are laid out in percentages and then converted into grams even for liquids, but so as not to blow the mathematical mind, we've kept it super simple – also avoiding you having to buy a .000 precise scale, which can be $$$.

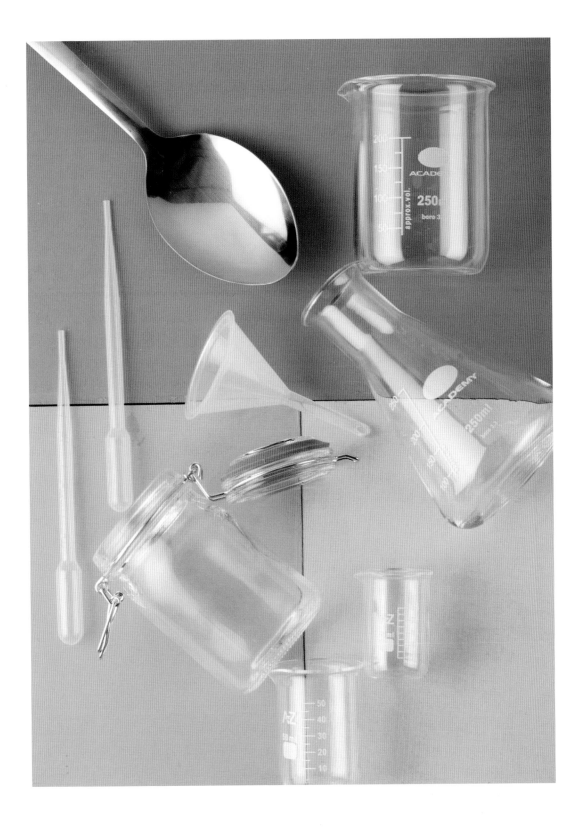

where the magic happens: how we formulate products

We like to take a fairly basic approach when formulating our products; we want our recipes to be simple, accessible and most of all fun for you all to try. As you'll see over the next few pages, including water can be complicated in any recipe that you'd like to have a decent shelf life and don't plan on using straight away. You'll therefore see that many of our 'DIY Beauty' recipes are anhydrous – that is, they contain no water. These are predominantly oil-based recipes that are incredibly easy to formulate and, on the whole, are made up of two key ingredients:

• Essential oils are the fragrant, highly concentrated oils derived from the external matter of a plant, such as the petals. We love using them as they are highly beneficial for skin and hair, as well as being linked to holistic, mental and general health. Essential oils are also a fantastic way to fragrance your recipes without having to use synthetic perfumes.

• Carrier oils are best known to you and me as vegetable, nut and seed oils. They tend to derive from the fatty part of a plant. They are much less potent than essential oils, and can therefore be used directly on the skin. They are called 'carrier oils' because their job is literally to carry the essential oil to the skin. Although not as strong, carrier oils are still hugely beneficial in their own right and are often used without the addition of an essential oil.

Simply using a combination of essential and carrier oils can create a highly effective product that takes on liquid form – this includes serums, cleansers, body oils, hair oils and so on. It is also possible to experiment with the texture of your products without needing to add water. Experimenting with different types of carrier oils is a good way to start – coconut oil is much firmer in its natural state than, say, olive oil, so will give you a much thicker texture. It's also important to see which carrier oil works best for your skin. You'll see that we use a number of other carrier products throughout the book, which result in products with a range of consistencies. Butters and beeswax, for instance, will lend a cream-like texture to your product without the need for a scientific process.

As you learn what oils your skin loves, and what textures work well for you, we encourage you to start mixing things up and customising recipes, always adhering to the foundations set out over the next few pages.

> **WARNING: Essential oils are highly potent and can be dangerous if used directly on the skin. Please read the section on Essential Oils, p. 22, before you begin to use them.**

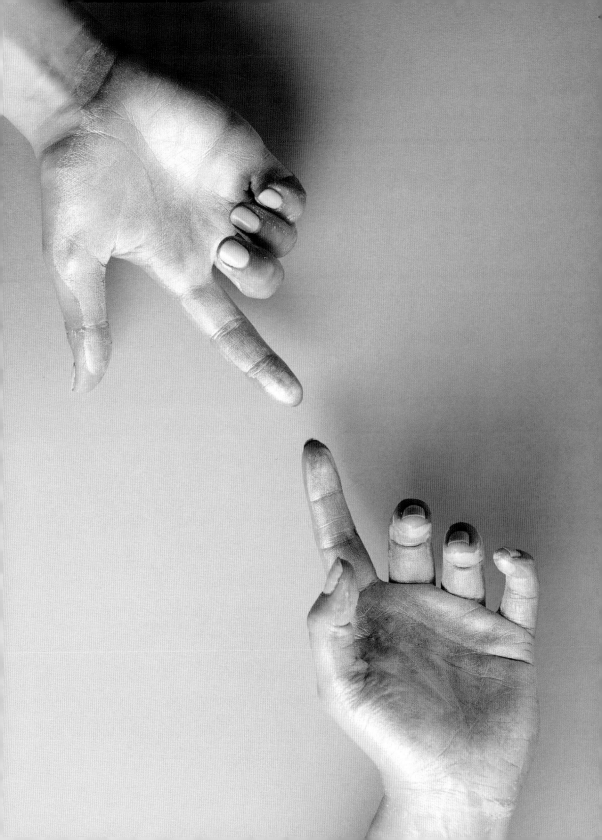

Beauty foundations you mix with

WATER

Take a quick look over the labels of a few of your favourite lotions and creams. One of the first ingredients is water, right? Right. Many brands like to cut corners: they shout about a product having a particular ingredient because they know that it's got beneficial properties, but then they only put 0.1 per cent of it into the finished product. Unfortunately, producers don't have to put ingredient percentages on packaging, so we never really know the true quantities of each ingredient, allowing manufacturers to heavily dilute their products while we remain none the wiser. Our only indicator is the fact that cosmetic labels read from high to low: the first ingredient is used the most and the last the least. Ever wondered why water appears as the first ingredient on your lotions, face washes, expensive eye creams? Yep, because there's a hell of lot of water in your products, sometimes up to 80 per cent. And you guessed it, water is cheap. It also has basically no beneficial properties for the skin.

The trouble is, once water is present, bacteria can grow. When not treated, this can lead to products becoming infested with yeast, mould and fungi. The ramifications of this are skin sensitivities, rashes and severe infections. There is an easy way to overcome this: the addition of a preservative will halt the growth of any bacteria and prolong the shelf life of a product. However, natural preservatives are expensive and so (you've guessed it) the big companies wind up using cheap and nasty alternatives.

So when we decided to make our own products, we actively chose to avoid water where possible. Instead, we use highly concentrated amounts of active ingredients that can actually have an effect; we're using natural, unprocessed ingredients; we're using less and wasting less. Oil-based and anhydrous products are easy to make as you don't need a science degree to formulate them. They are safe, don't need preserving, and it's pretty difficult to go wrong.

But there are some ingredients that are beneficial for the skin, but do contain water – things like aloe vera, floral waters, milk, fresh fruit and vegetables. So the absolute golden rule is: if water is present, you must always use a preservative. We've included a section in the FAQs about natural preservatives and some

101 — what can what and why?

accessible ones to begin experimenting with (see p. 211). Suppliers tend to sell aloe vera and floral waters pre-preserved so they've done the hard work for you. Just be sure to check with the supplier before you buy. We'll call out shelf lives for you throughout the recipes; for anything that you can't buy pre-preserved (i.e. fresh fruit and veg), you need to store in the fridge and use within a week.

OIL AND WATER

Remember those groovy lava lamps everyone wanted at school? They taught us all that oil and water don't mix when combined alone. The only way to disperse oil into water is to use an emulsifier, i.e. a chemical used to stabilise the emulsion of oil and water. The process can be tricky because it involves a lot of precise heating and cooling, so we've avoided that where possible in this book. The big corporations love working with (often cheap) emulsifiers to blend oil and water – diluting the potency of the oil, meaning they can use less but end up with more of the finished product. We believe you can achieve a creamy texture without using any water at all – many oil-based ingredients will do the job just as well.

Having said all this, sometimes we do like to blend this dynamic duo – with fantastic results – but there are just a couple of things to remember.

Essential oils only disperse if placed in another oil and essential oils shouldn't be used directly on the skin. You therefore can't put essential oils directly into water that is going to be used to the skin, for example in a bath or in a floral water. You run the risk of burning or irritating your skin. If you want to put essential oils into water, you need to add the essential oil with an ingredient that mixes with water, such as Epsom salts, milk powders or oats, or disperse into a carrier oil first.

You must also bear in mind that your mixture won't look quite as you imagined if you've used water and oil without an emulsifier. An example of this is our Micellar Water (p. 128). You'll notice that the carrier oil floats around the mixture in large blobs, but we quite dig this look! If you shake well before spraying you'll still get an even distribution of oil and water, plus it's safe to use this way as the carrier oil isn't as potent as the essential oil (see Essential Oils: Safety First p. 20).

burn, baby, burn

When heating butters, waxes and oils, it is advisable to do so in a bain-marie. This is a bowl, sitting over a pan of water which is over heat (i.e. on a hob), so that it gently heats without burning. We do this in cooking sometimes, like when melting chocolate (yuuuum-o) so the mixture melts evenly and at a low heat. It's important in beauty because ingredients can quickly lose their nutritional value when exposed to high temperatures. Essential oils also evaporate at high temperatures, so always add these once your mixture has cooled.

hygiene

We've saved the most important bit 'til last. We are firm believers that you should approach your beauty making in the same way that you approach food preparation. Would you stir your soup with a dirty spoon? Cut your veggies on a chopping board that hasn't been washed? Eat a piece of rotten fruit? Thought not. The same applies to beauty. Basically, if your recipe is subject to any bacteria, or any conditions in which bacteria can grow, it will go off. Rancid products can cause skin reactions, allergies, rashes and irritation, which is not quite the dewy glow that one would hope for. They will also just not work as well as a fresh recipe. We have to be strict with this one, it's only because we want the best for you guys. Here are the key points to follow: we promise they aren't too tricky.

• Make sure any tools or surfaces you are using have been sterilised before you use them. We don't expect you to invest in a brand-new set of kit specifically for beauty; it's fine to use your kitchen essentials. Just please make sure they have been cleaned in the dishwasher and then again in boiling water between uses.

• It's absolutely fine to recycle your existing containers; just ensure your containers are clean (again in the dishwasher and sterilised with boiling water) and <u>DRY</u>. We emphasise this because using containers that still have a little water in them is exactly the same as adding water to your mixture and, yup, you guessed it, water = bacteria growth.

• Finally, invest in a good apron, hairnets and disposable gloves. This one isn't essential if you're whipping up a quick face mask but we think it's good practice, particularly if you're making products in bulk or as gifts. Plus everyone looks fabulous in a hairnet.

PATCH TEST

When applying anything new to the skin, it's important to sense check that your skin doesn't react negatively. While this is unlikely in the ingredients we've chosen, you may have underlying allergies that you've not been made aware of. As best practise, patch test any new products on an indiscreet area of the body (we love an elbow or ankle) prior to applying to the face or sensitive body parts. If everything is dandy after 24 hours, go ahead and commence slathering.

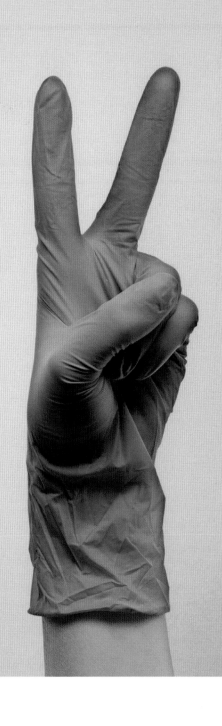

Essential oils: safety first!

You probably guessed this by now, but we love essential oils. Their potency, fragrance and benefits for the body both inside and out make them unlike any other ingredient in formulation. They are incredibly multi-talented. Take lavender, for example: it's linked to soothing inflamed skin and is often used in the treatment of eczema. But it also has wonderful calming properties for the mind and can be used to treat insomnia. Pretty amazing for a tiny bottle of liquid, huh?

Essential oils are fragrant and highly concentrated liquids typically extracted from a plant's leaves, berries, grasses, flowering tops, petals, roots, zest, resin and wood. Their powerful properties are down to the fact that they are incredibly potent; the process of extracting the oil requires an extremely high quantity of the source plant matter to produce a very small quantity of oil. In that small quantity will be a huge amount of the herb or flower in question, much more than any carrier oil, hydrosol (see p. 24 for the 411 on hydrosols) or butter. To put it into perspective, it takes about 150kg of lavender to produce 1kg of oil.

What that means for us is that because these oils are so powerful, there are a number of safety rules you MUST follow whilst handling them. Failure to do so could result in skin irritation, reactions, rashes or burning. Even the toughest of skin will find 150kg of lavender a lot to cope with! Read this section thoroughly before you start to use essential oils.

1   Never use directly on the skin. We've talked about the job of a carrier oil – to act as an enabler for your essential oil, meaning you're able to use it in your products. The intensity of the essential oil is too much for many people's skin to cope with and could result in unwanted reactions such as burning. Your essential oil must be diluted in an oil, butter, wax, salt, or other oil-soluble carrier product. You may read contradictory advice about certain essential oils such as tea tree or lavender, suggesting that they're suitable to be used directly on the skin. In order to avoid confusion, we apply the same golden rule to all essential oils.

2   Keep that golden rule in mind when you are handing essential oils: never let them come into contact with your skin; better still, wear disposable gloves.

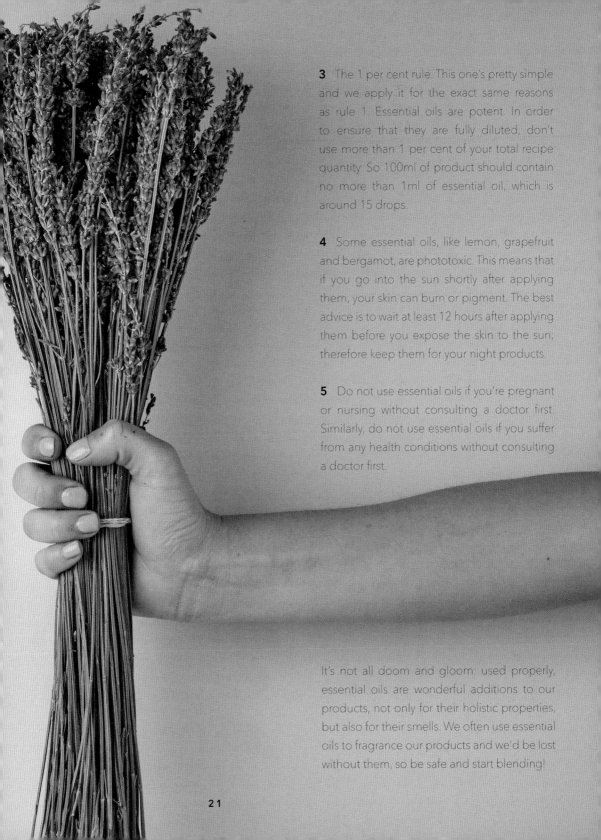

3 The 1 per cent rule. This one's pretty simple and we apply it for the exact same reasons as rule 1. Essential oils are potent. In order to ensure that they are fully diluted, don't use more than 1 per cent of your total recipe quantity. So 100ml of product should contain no more than 1ml of essential oil, which is around 15 drops.

4 Some essential oils, like lemon, grapefruit and bergamot, are phototoxic. This means that if you go into the sun shortly after applying them, your skin can burn or pigment. The best advice is to wait at least 12 hours after applying them before you expose the skin to the sun; therefore keep them for your night products.

5 Do not use essential oils if you're pregnant or nursing without consulting a doctor first. Similarly, do not use essential oils if you suffer from any health conditions without consulting a doctor first.

It's not all doom and gloom: used properly, essential oils are wonderful additions to our products, not only for their holistic properties, but also for their smells. We often use essential oils to fragrance our products and we'd be lost without them, so be safe and start blending!

a 101 on natural ingredients
carrier oils:

Carrier oils are the base of many recipes in this book and will usually make up the highest proportion of the ingredients list. They derive from the fatty portion of a plant, usually from the seeds, kernels or the nuts, and their purpose is to dilute essential oils or carry them onto the skin. Carriers have a number of benefits in their own right, though, and can be used directly on skin or hair. It's best to buy organic oils, which ensures the plant hasn't been exposed to pesticides and other chemicals, and cold-pressed where possible, as this means they haven't been heated during processing, which destroys some of the nutrients. Here are our faves.

Apricot Kernel Oil	Quickly absorbed, making it ideal to use on the face; high in vitamin A, which is linked to prolonging collagen production, so an ideal anti-ager.
Argan Oil	Helps to balance the levels of sebum (the natural oil your skin produces), which in turn fights acne and spots. Incredibly high vitamin E levels make it a great non-greasy hair treatment.
Avocado Oil	High in essential fatty acids, which means it's ultra-nourishing and moisturising; best for dry skin.
Baobab Oil	Comes from the Anansonia tree, which absorbs and retains water during the rainy season to replenish itself during the dry months. This tree can live for up to 1500 years. Seriously, if that doesn't sound like an enticing beauty proposition, we don't know what does! Rich in Vitamin E and free radical fighting anti-oxidants.
Castor Oil	A thick, sticky oil not commonly used as a carrier oil. It's a highly effective emollient, preventing water loss from the skin, and its naturally thick consistency means it's fab for hair shine.
Coconut Oil	All-round superstar, we literally use this stuff for everything. It's high in medium-chain fatty acids, which penetrate the skin deeply and lock in moisture. See p. 52 for more coco love.

Evening Primrose Oil	This herb contains a high concentration of a fatty acid called GLA; it is this fatty acid that is largely responsible for the remarkable healing properties of the plant. Great for anti-ageing and healing products.
Grapeseed Oil	A great source of polyphenols, flavonoids, linoleic acid and vitamin E, all potent antioxidants. It's also cost effective and typically used in massage oils and wash-off products.
Jojoba Oil	Lightweight and versatile, it closely resembles human sebum and therefore helps balance out oily skin.
Macadamia Nut Oil	Expressed directly from the nut, this oil contains a high level of antioxidants including the rarer tocotrienols (found in vitamin E); it's also super light and fast absorbing.
Olive Oil	Heavy and super moisturising, this one's ideal for dry skin or using at night. Great in hair treatments and also good as an alternative carrier for anyone with nut allergies.
Pomegranate Seed Oil	Obtained from cold-pressing the fruit seed, the oil contains a unique polyunsaturated oil, punicic acid, an omega-5 fatty acid, which has strong anti-inflammatory properties and is also high in antioxidants.
Prickly Pear Oil (aka Barbary Fig Oil)	Derived from the small cactus plant, this is a rich oil great for ageing skin due to its linoleic acid content, which helps to stimulate cell growth and to fight free radicals (flip to p. 40 to find out why we're not fans of free radicals). Expensive but worth it, trust us.
Rosehip Oil	Astringent properties and essential fatty acids make this fab for stretch marks, pigmentation and cellulite. A natural source of vitamin C that brightens the skin.
Sweet Almond Oil	High in vitamin A, so it's a great anti-inflammatory and will help soothe red, irritated or flaky skin. Also great for dark under-eye circles.

hydrosols:

Hydrosols – also known as floral waters, hydrolats, flower waters or distillates – are derived from the water collected when plants are steamed for their essential oils. This light, fragrant water holds similar benefits to its respective essential oil, but without the same level of potency. This means hydrosols can be used directly on the skin and hair. They are also used to fragrance a product. We always recommend buying pre-preserved hydrosols as they are still water based. See the FAQs on p. 211 for details of our fave stockists.

Chamomile Hydrosol	Chamomile is incredibly soothing with fantastic anti-inflammatory properties. We use it to calm tired, sore or irritated skin and for sunburn. It has a delicate floral scent, so mixes well with other hydrosols, and is perfect for an all-over body spritz.
Lavender Hydrosol	Its scent makes it an ideal bedtime toner to aid sleep, a lovely addition to a relaxing bath or a nice room spray. Lavender has been linked with the healing of skin conditions such as eczema due to its anti-inflammatory and soothing properties, so this is a nice option for those with sensitive skin.
Orange Blossom Hydrosol	Deriving from the bitter orange tree, orange blossom hydrosol is great for tightening and brightening skin, with rejuvenating properties making it the ideal facial toner or spritz. It has a strong scent so it's also good when used as a perfume.
Peppermint Hydrosol	A heavily scented hydrosol that is both refreshing and uplifting. Great antibacterial and antimicrobial properties make it an ideal mouthwash, cleanser, toner, foot spray or deodorant.
Rose Hydrosol	Often associated with anti-ageing products due to its astringent properties and ability to have a tightening effect on mature skin. Rosewater is also high in vitamins A and B, so provides a great nutrient boost whilst hydrating. Perfect for toners, face masks, deodorants, foot sprays, body sprays and hair treatments.
Witch Hazel	Often used in the treatment of spots, skin conditions, bruises and wounds, witch hazel has fabulous healing properties, is anti-inflammatory, antibacterial and a great astringent.

butters:

Butters are extracted from the fattiest part of the plant, often the seed or stone, and are thick, hard and stable in consistency. This makes them perfect for creating a lotion- or cream-type texture, without needing the addition of water, emollients or emulsifiers. Butters usually need melting down before you begin working with them but once they're in liquid form, mix them as you would any other carrier oils. We love experimenting with textures; changing the ratio of butter to oil is a great way to do this, or whipping the butter when it's liquid. Always opt for unrefined and organic options. These are our faves.

Cocoa Butter	Difficult not to love anything so closely related to our all-time favourite comfort food. Deriving from the cacao bean, this butter is also edible and smells delightful, so it's perfect if you're looking to fragrance a product. Ideal for use on all skin types and super moisturising.
Mango Butter	Derived from the mango seed, mango butter has a slightly firmer consistency than other butters due to its higher melting point. As a result, it makes a great base for thicker products (body butters, lip balms, etc.). Its high content of vitamin E means it's a powerful antioxidant, so good for more mature skin. Its fatty acid levels help promote elasticity. Use it in smaller quantities due to its dense texture.
Muru Muru Butter	Extracted from the fatty part of the muru muru palm tree seed and grown natively in the Brazilian Amazon region. It's an incredibly nourishing butter: highly emollient with a glossy sheen, and has a high content of omega-9 rich oleic acid. Muru muru butter works wonderfully in body butters but it's also beneficial for the hair, softening and protecting it. This makes it a great addition to any hair waxes, beard balms and treatments.
Shea Butter	Extracted from the shea nut of the karité tree, this is a rich, nourishing and moisturising butter ideal for dry or flaky skin. It is also used to help with stretch marks, scars and skin conditions due to its amazing healing abilities. It melts at body temperature so, despite its thick consistency, it glides on easily to skin, making it ideal for both the body and the face.

essential oils:

Carrot Seed Oil	Strong antioxidant properties and incredibly detoxifying, this is great for cleansing and purifying all skin types whilst being super hydrating.
Frankincense Oil	An anti-ageing hero that helps tighten skin and reduce the appearance of wrinkles. It's also got a lovely smell, so it's good as a natural fragrance.
Geranium Oil	Balances oil production, so great for spots and suitable for all skin types. Smells delightful.
Grapefruit Oil	Astringent and high in antioxidants that help stimulate blood flow, in turn remedying lumps, bumps and cellulite (YES, cellulite).
Lavender Oil	Antiseptic and anti-inflammatory properties make it a good remedy for acne, eczema and other skin problems; it is also soothing and calming for the muscles and the mind.
Neroli Oil	Emollient properties lock in moisture to the skin. Regenerates skin elasticity, which makes it a firm fave in anti-ageing or rejuvenating products but it does come with a pretty hefty price tag.
Patchouli Oil	Antiseptic and rich, so great for moisturising particularly dry skin. This one has a deep, manly scent.
Rose Absolute Oil	Anti-inflammatory, which makes it great for sensitive skin types. Well known for smoothing ageing skin, nourishing, moisturising and being an all-round superstar. Used at a maximum of 0.2 per cent for leave-on products.
Tea Tree Oil	Powerful antiseptic and antibacterial properties; it's ideal for acne, skin conditions and fungal problems.

and finally, the rest of the gang:

Aloe Vera

Deriving directly from the leaves of the aloe vera plant, this gel-like substance is a miracle worker. It is a fantastic healer due to its antibacterial and anti-inflammatory properties, but also perfect for skin cell rejuvenation thanks to its antioxidant powers. It is often used directly on sunburn, wounds, eczema or psoriasis; we also love adding it to oils or waters to provide a gel-like consistency. Always buy pre-preserved or use in powdered form.

Beeswax

Produced by honeybees in the hive and therefore not suitable if you are a strict vegan. It instantly provides a balm-like texture when mixed with oils, even if used in small quantities. It produces a film over the top layer of skin so is great at protecting against the elements in products like lip balms, and is also used to firm and nourish. We find grated beeswax easiest to work with. Once heated, it cools and hardens very quickly so it's best to mix with oils whilst still on a low heat. Candelilla wax is a great vegan alternative.

Clay

These are natural fine-grained rock or soil minerals that are ultra-absorbing. Clay can bind molecules to the surface, mineralising and detoxifying the skin. Different colours have different properties: white kaolin and pink clays are great for sensitive skin, the darker clays like rhassoul and green have the most absorbent properties, making them great for oily skin (and hair!).

Dr Bronner's Castile Soap

OK, so technically this isn't a raw ingredient, but it's so useful we had to give old Bronner a shout-out. It is a liquid soap made out of natural ingredients – coconut, jojoba, hemp and palm kernel – and gently foams when lathered. It's a great base for expanding out into shampoos and body washes without going through the complications of emulsifiers and surfactants (chemical compounds that create foam). You can get it unscented or naturally scented.

Glycerine

This is a natural constituent of fatty acid triglycerides and is often used in water-based products for its humectant (moisture-retaining) properties. It has a gel-like consistency, which makes it great for thickening.

Skin school

Sharpen those pencils and grab your note-pads, we're heading back to school. Before we set off, we want to go over some of the basics when it comes to your skin. It might not make your pub chat better (in fact it won't), but it will definitely make you understand the best ingredients for your skin.

Some interesting facts about our skin:

1 The skin is the body's largest organ. It weighs, on average, around 4kg and is about 2 square metres in size. Seriously impressive and definitely something that needs our care and attention!

2 The skin sheds about 30,000 to 40,000 dead cells per minute.

3 The thinnest layer of skin is around the eyes and the thickest is the palms of our hands and the heels of our feet. And that explains why you need to be super-careful about using non-irritating ingredients around the eye area.

4 Our skin regulates body temperature by detecting hot and cold.

5 Every square inch of the skin holds 300 sweat glands. But sweat doesn't actually smell – it's the reaction between the bacteria that naturally sits on the skin and the sweat that causes an odour.

Your skin is comprised of two main layers: the epidermis, the outer skin, and the dermis, the inner skin, and has several layers within each dermis. The layer most impacted by cosmetics is the *stratum corneum*, or the horny layer (naughty) and age affects how quickly this layer is replaced, in a process called desquamation. In younger skin it can take 14 days and older skin can take up to 37. The skin completely renews itself after 28 days. This is an important fact to remember when testing a new product or routine: it will take a minimum of 14 days for the product to really show its impact and up to 28 for the full effect to become clear. The performance and reaction of the skin is incredibly unique to individuals, and one size truly does not fit all. When you make one of these recipes for the first time, always patch test it on an area of skin before applying all over.

One way of deciding, and analysing an oil's benefit to the skin is its comedogenic rating. In DIY-babe language, this means how likely an oil is to clog your pores. Coconut oil rates highly on this scale; it's an occlusive oil that forms a thick layer on the top of your skin and doesn't let anything in or out. This sounds like a bit of a nightmare, but if you have super dry skin as a result of eczema, you want to lock in moisture and keep drying environmental elements out. If you have acne-prone skin, however, you should avoid using a comedogenic oil on your face, as this can lead to breakouts. At the other end of the scale, there are light oils like jojoba or apricot. Their compounds compliment the skin's natural state. These are great for oily and blemish-prone skins as they balance the skin's pH. Keep the comedogenic rating in mind when you're formulating — always choose ingredients that are right for your skin type.

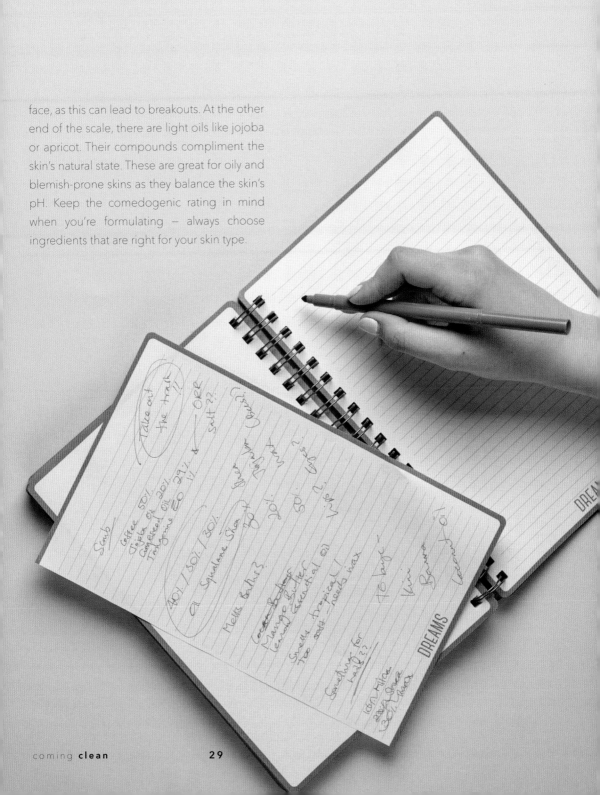

7 *Steps to* Going Clean

1. Understand what's in your existing products

Do a little research and let what you find do the talking. There are a ton of ingredients used only to prolong a shelf life, to pad out a product, to make it smell nice, to make it lather or give it that cream-like consistency. Some of these ingredients have even been accused of causing damage to our health. While there is still heated debate within the scientific and cosmetic communities on many of these, we're of the minds that if there's a risk, why take the chance? Do the research and you'll soon understand why clean beauty is so important. Recommended reading: *Not Just a Pretty Face* by Stacy Malkan; *No More Dirty Looks* by Siobhan O'Connor & Alexandra Spunt.

2. Know where to start

Don't freak out. We know that's likely to be your gut reaction, because we experienced exactly the same thing. Feeling as if you've been cheated by your favourite brands for all these years. You trusted them! And now all you want to do is go running into your bathroom with a blowtorch and incinerate every last trace of your traitor products. Well, just hold your horses for one second. Whist very tempting, that isn't a great idea on a number of levels (it's a fire hazard for a start), the main one being that it's an incredibly expensive and time-consuming process to replace your face cream, shower gel, shampoo, conditioner, serum, body scrub… It'd take you weeks to make the lot from scratch or cost you hundreds to buy brand-new, non-toxic replacements for every product all at once. So instead we say this: be smart and know where to start. Your body. We've discussed the fact that your skin absorbs much of what's put on it and that it's the biggest organ of your body. So it makes sense to firstly minimise the largest area of exposure to potential toxins. You can make a couple of simple changes to your body's beauty regime without spending loads, and drastically reduce your exposure to dirty products. Focus on switching your body wash and creams as a starting point, then move onto your face and hair once you've nailed that.

3. One product at a time

We guarantee that once you start, you won't be able to stop. Replacing your products is incredibly satisfying and you'll be feeling pretty smug. It's addictive and the temptation is to spend a weekend locked in the kitchen like a mad scientist, only emerging once you've made every single recipe in the *Clean Beauty* book. Focus on one product at a time. There are two key reasons for this:

a) You may find that some are more effective than others but will have absolutely no idea which. How do you know what's giving you that youthful glow? Is it your brand-new rose toner or your face scrub? Not one body is the same and whilst a coffee body scrub will work wonders for many, others may find that their skin doesn't take particularly well to it. The best way to attack your new routine is one product at a time.

b) It's bloody expensive.

Firstly replace your shower gel, find a new alternative that your skin loves, then move onto your moisturiser, scrub, and so on. Particularly when you get to your face and new cosmetics, you'll find things so much more manageable if your focus is on just one product.

---

4. Expect the unexpected

Your skin has been used to a certain type of product for many years. It will include pointless fillers, which hold little nutritional value, and a great deal of water and it is also unlikely to have the potency of pure, unprocessed ingredients in any large quantities. You may go from using a face serum with 0.5 per cent rosehip oil to making your very own with 80 per cent rosehip and that initial, high-intensity hit of nutrients may be shocking to the skin. Be prepared for breakouts – your skin's way of expelling existing toxins. Stick it out for a few days, because nine times out of ten your body adjusts and ends up loving the absolute potency approach.

Disclaimer: please stop using a product if the reaction is sore, itchy, inflamed or becomes any kind of rash. It's likely that you're intolerant to an ingredient if such a reaction occurs (and if you're tackling one product at a time, you should easily be able to trace the cause of this). This also where a patch test becomes important (see p. 18).

5. Don't beat yourself up

Going green is a lifestyle change. It's a long process. It takes effort. It's incredibly rewarding but we certainly admit that you're kicking the habits of a lifetime. So don't beat yourself up. Fnish that super-expensive Mac foundation rather than just chucking it out. Don't feel bad if you use the shower gel in the gym because you have no alternative, or a spritz of deodorant from a mate as you have nothing on you and you absolutely stink. Clean beauty is a holistic approach to a better beauty regime, but we know that, because of the society that we live in, it's not always possible to find an easy and non-toxic alternative to a product that's otherwise widely available. Be proud of your progress and take a healthy and realistic approach to your routine.

---

6. Get creative

Once you've got started on the recipes you'll soon get a good idea of your favourites. Then you're free to get creative and go a little off-piste with your recipe creation. This is an entry-level guide to DIY beauty but most of our recipes are customisable in some way. Once you begin to recognise yourself as the green beauty guru that you are, you gotta unleash your creative juices in the kitchen. You'll soon know which butters your skin loves, which essential oils make you smell like a babe and which carrier oils give you total goddess hair. So put that knowledge to good use and become the next Clean Beauty Co.

Don't forget that we LOVE hearing about your concoctions, so please share your creations with us over Instagram with the hashtag #cleanbeautycrew – we regularly regram our favourites.

7.
Enjoy it!

DIY beauty is empowering and gives you the chance to take control over what you put on your skin. It's an exciting journey and we're so glad that you're joining us on it! So have fun with it! Tell your mates! And welcome to the crew.

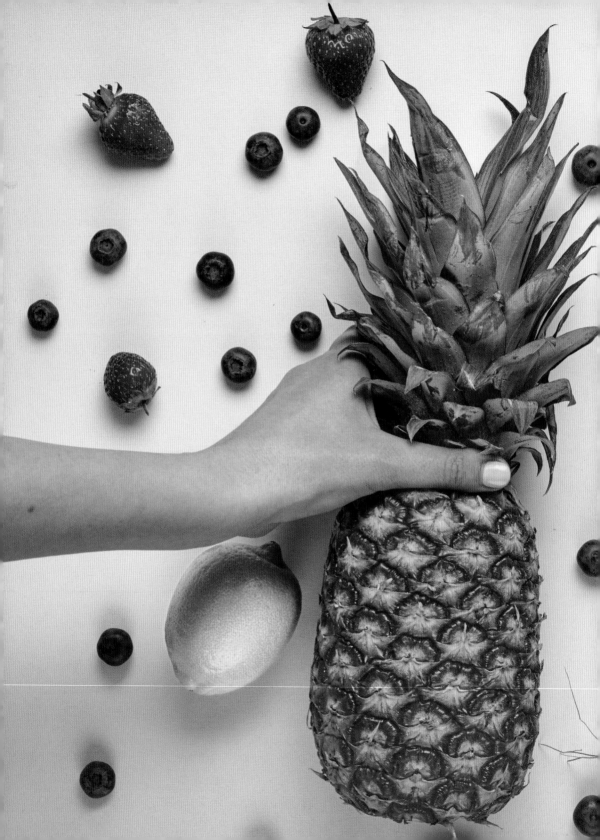

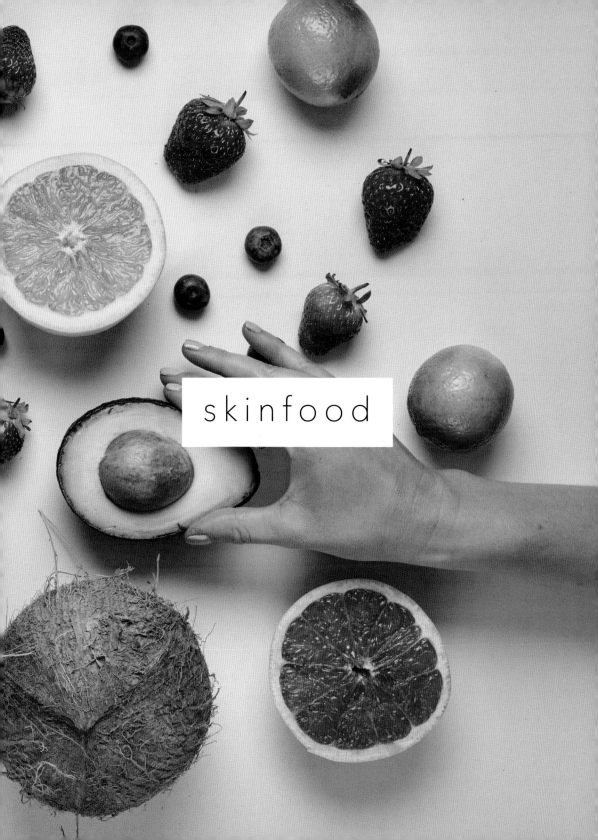

skinfood

Great skin starts in the kitchen. We are firm believers that if it's good enough to go in your smoothie, it's sure as hell good enough to slather all over your face. In *Skinfood*, you'll find a compilation of our very best tried and tested recipes made using just your kitchen essentials.

face

face detox

1 tablespoon kaolin clay
1 tablespoon yogurt
1 teaspoon spirulina

MAKES:
One mask

SHELF LIFE:
Immediate use; store in the fridge for up to 3 days.

HELPFUL HINT:
You can replace the yogurt with milk or kefir, or coconut yogurt if vegan.

This face mask is a simple blend of three ingredients but wow, does it make you glow! Kaolin clay is one of the most commonly available and versatile cosmetic clays, as it has a high mineral content, gentle nature and absorbent properties. Yogurt contains lactic acid, a beta hydroxy acid that acts as a gentle exfoliator, removing dead skin cells and leaving skin soft and smooth. Spirulina has a high content of vitamins A, B12 and E, so it can improve sagging, tired-looking skin, promoting a more youthful, radiant complexion, and fight ageing free radicals. It also stimulates epidermal growth and repair. Apply this after a big night out to feel human again!

---

1 Mix all the ingredients together.
2 Apply to the face.
3 Leave until the clay is dry and the skin feels tight.
4 Remove with a warm wet cloth.

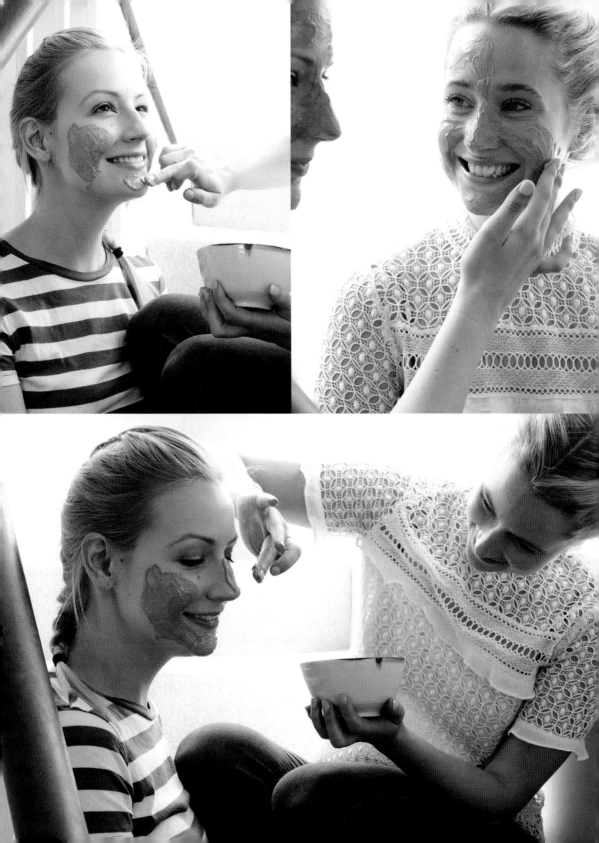

What's up with *free radicals?*

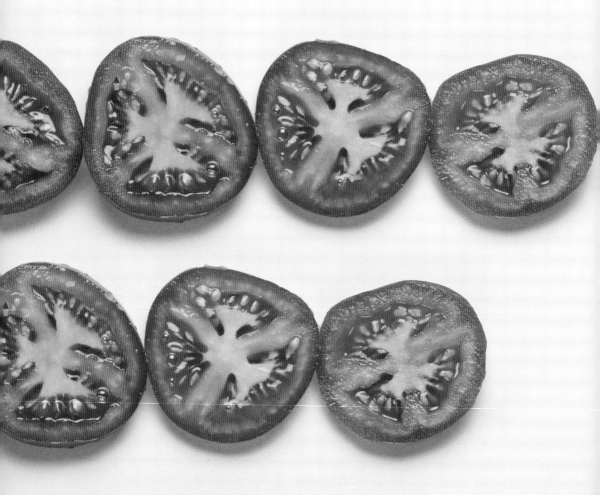

these

Throughout the book we talk a lot about free radicals, but what exactly are they and why do we want to work against them in skincare?

We are all made up of millions of microscopic molecules: clever little cells that work hard to keep us healthy. Free radicals are molecules that become unstable and radicalised when damaged – by the environment, UV rays or pollution, for example. The unstable cell will instinctively try to repair itself, usually by bonding on to the nearest healthy cell to gain stability. This in turn damages the healthy cell, which then latches onto another healthy cell, and the process of destabilisation continues. This is known as the free radical chain and, over time, the damage that free radicals cause becomes visible on the skin, particularly on the face and neck. The process of cell radicalisation happens naturally as we get old (dammit!) but it is also proliferated by environmental factors such as chemicals and pollution, UV rays and smoking. The free radical theory of ageing suggests that free radical damage is actually the cause of all visible ageing. The combined effects of age, metabolism and the environment make cells weaker and more susceptible to damage, so we end up with wrinkles, fine lines, age spots and loose skin. Boo, you free radicals!

So naturally, we want to stop these ageing radicals in their tracks. We need to offer these damaged cells something they can use to repair themselves, in order to halt the formation of further free radical chains. Antioxidants, like vitamins C and E, have been proven to help stabilise damaged molecules and stop any further cellular damage. In order to get an antioxidant boost, consume foods rich in vitamin C, such as tomatoes, oranges and spinach, or get your vitamin E from plant oils, almonds and sunflower seeds. Notice we include antioxidants and antioxidant-rich ingredients a lot in our recipes. Makes sense, right? Right.

fragrant face bronzer

1 teaspoon ground cinnamon
1 teaspoon cocoa powder
1 teaspoon ground nutmeg
2 teaspoons arrowroot powder

Our take on the classic mineral bronzer uses ingredients from your spice drawer to give you that summer glow. Quantities are approximate based on colouring, so adjustment is needed depended on the shade desired. Cocoa gives depth and darkness, so is not imperative for lighter shades. Nutmeg and cinnamon create the warm brown glow, and arrowroot will ensure everything combines and spreads evenly.

MAKES:
15g

SHELF LIFE:
3 months; apply with a brush not fingers!

HELPFUL HINT:
You can add mica powder for a subtle shimmer.

1 Mix the powders well in a small bowl, breaking up any clumps.
2 Transfer to an empty make-up compact.
3 Use a brush to apply when needed.

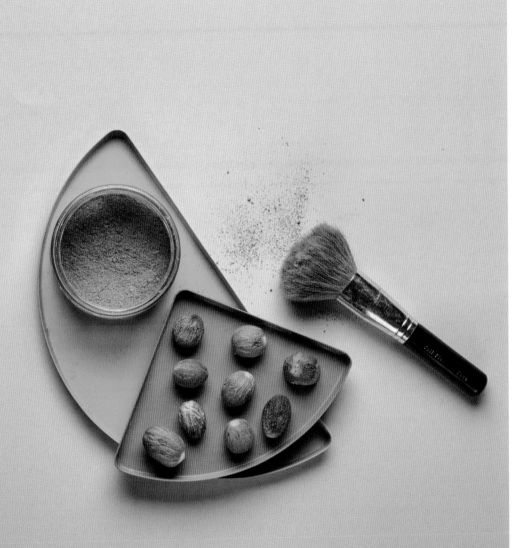

sweet botanicals toner

½ tablespoon honey

5 tablespoons filtered water

1 tablespoon apple cider vinegar

4 drops lavender essential oil

This is a skin-healing toner: gently antibacterial, promoting skin cell renewal and an even skin tone. It works best post-cleansing or as a make-up setter. Apple cider vinegar helps to balance the skin's pH levels, while lavender is regenerative and healing on the skin. This is a great, effective toner for all skin types.

1 Mix the ingredients together well.

2 Decant into a spray bottle.

3 Shake well before use.

4 Spray onto a clean, dry face and leave to absorb.

MAKES:
100ml

SHELF LIFE:
Up to 1 week in the fridge.

HELPFUL HINT:
You can spray this onto a cotton pad and use as a make-up remover as well.

oaty superfood cleanser

2 tablespoons oatmeal
1 teaspoon baobab
powder
4 tablespoons water

MAKES:
One use

SHELF LIFE:
One-time use.

HELPFUL HINT:
You could use any
superfood you have in
your kitchen: matcha for an
antioxidant hit; spirulina,
high in iron, to help improve
the skin's elasticity; or acai,
which is rich in vitamins A,
C and E, to help fight those
free radicals.

This one is super simple but it's as effective as anything you'll get on the high street, particularly for dry or sensitive skin. Soaking the oats prior to use turns the mixture into a lovely milky porridge to slather all over. Oats have traditionally been used to treat dry skin; they contain the avenanthramide class of antioxidants, which are effective anti-inflammatories reducing redness and also protecting the skin against UV sun damage. In this instance, we're using oatmeal as the ground oats give a great texture to the cleanser. While baobab oil can be harder to obtain, the chances are you have a sachet or two of the powder lying around for smoothies. The nutrients in baobab improve skin elasticity and complexion restoration, rich as it is in vitamins A, D, E and F. The mixture will cleanse and nourish the skin, removing dirt and grime after a day in the city.

---

1 Mix the ingredients together and leave for 30 minutes prior to use.
2 Use as a normal cleanser, rubbing in circular motions.
3 Wash off with warm water.

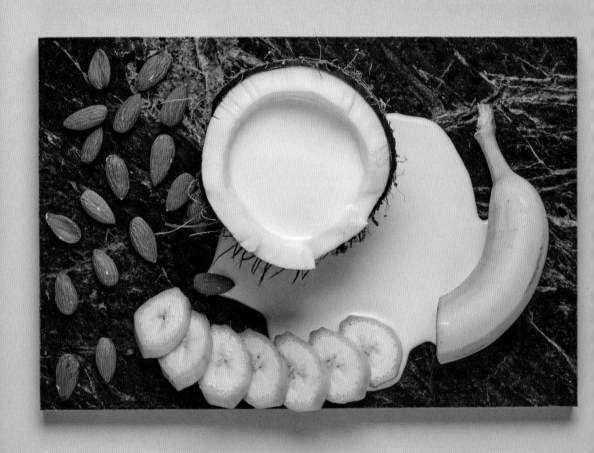

banana bread

½ ripe banana, mashed
1 tablespoon ground
   almonds
1 tablespoon coconut
   milk

MAKES:
One use

SHELF LIFE:
One-time use.

HELPFUL HINT:
You could switch the
coconut milk for regular
milk or yogurt.

A quick peep at this and you might be expecting to make a delicious baked goodie – but no, this one's for your face. Bananas are rich in potassium and vitamins A, B and E, which promote moisture retention, even out skin tone and protect the skin against free radicals. Ground almonds are a great natural exfoliant, gently sweeping away dead skin cells and leaving you glowing. Nourishing coconut milk is a great addition to this scrub: it has all the benefits of coconut oil, but it's non-occlusive unlike its oil counterpart, which means that it doesn't block your pores and lets your skin breathe. Coconut milk is also a great make-up remover!

---

1 Mix all the ingredients into a paste.
2 Use as a scrub on the face, washing off once cleansed.

flawless face lift

¼ avocado, mashed
1 tablespoon honey
1 teaspoon matcha
   powder

MAKES:
One use

SHELF LIFE:
One-time use; store in the
fridge for up to 1 week.

HELPFUL HINT:
You could add protein-rich
whisked egg whites to give
your skin extra tightness
and lift but it will need to be
used immediately.

We all know about the benefits of the avocado for the body:
it is an unusually oily fruit and a rich source of vitamins A
and E. It is particularly beneficial to skin due to its antioxidant
and collagen-boosting properties. Matcha tea further enhances
the antioxidising benefits of the mix. In fact, the potent powder
has thirty-six times the antioxidants found in green tea. It's also
a good source of chlorophyll and catechins, compounds that
fight free radical damage and inflammation. Honey is rich in
antibacterial properties that help fight breakouts, acne and skin
imperfections. It also tastes delicious, so if you have any leftovers, send them our way, we're feeling peckish!

---

1 Mix all the ingredients into a smooth paste.
2 Place in the fridge to chill for 5 minutes.
3 Apply to the face and neck, leaving on for 5–10 minutes.

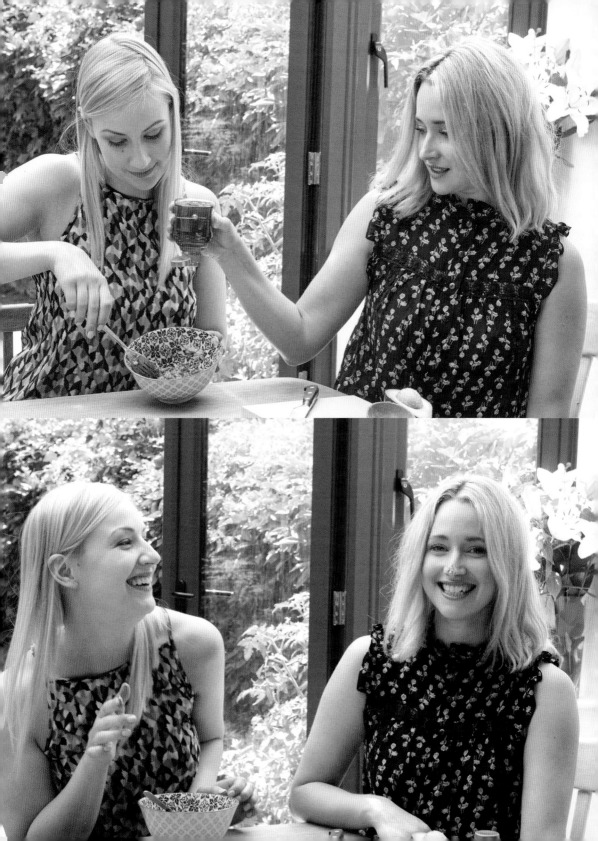

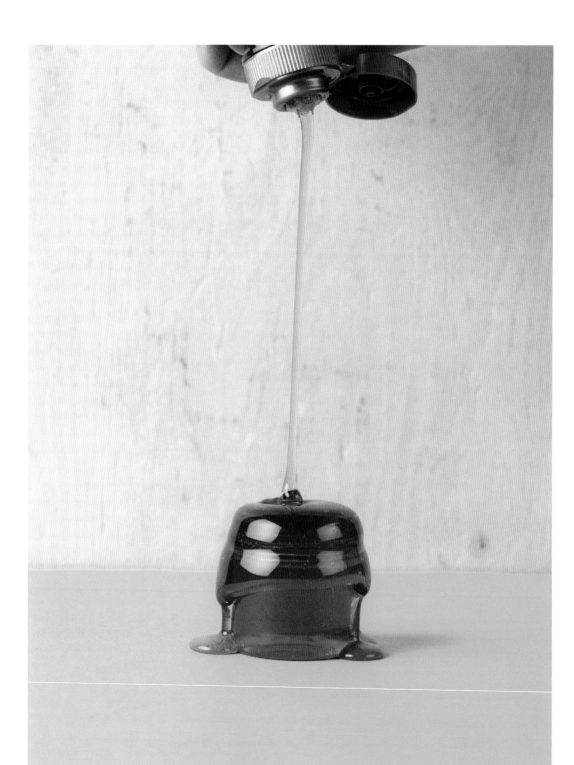

get your glow

2 tablespoons honey
1 tablespoon olive oil
10g ground almonds
1 tablespoon lemon juice

———————

MAKES:
One use

SHELF LIFE:
One-time use; store in the fridge for up to 1 week.

HELPFUL HINT:
Leave the lemon juice out if you've got sensitive skin.

Whip together this facial scrub to give that summer glow. Good-quality honey is antibacterial and rich in antioxidants, which is wonderful for the face to ensure blemish-free, glowing skin. See p. 106 for more on why we love honey. Ground almonds are gently abrasive, making them a great gentle exfoliator, and lemon is rich in AHAs, which help to gently peel away dead skin cells, revealing fresh skin underneath. Olive oil is anti-ageing; it is largely constructed of anti-oxidising vitamin E, which restores skin smoothness and protects against ultraviolet light. Hydroxytyrosol, a rare compound found in olive oil, prevents free radical damage to the skin. This baby is going to leave you gleaming. Can we get a whoop whoop?

———————

1 Blend the honey, lemon juice and olive oil.
2 Add the ground almonds to make a thick paste.
3 Gently scrub in circular motions on the face and wash off with warm water.

Loco *for the*

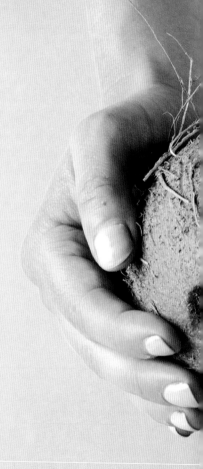

We bang on about coconut oil a lot. We're aware of that. But our buddy Coco so deserves it.

Coconut oil is the holy grail of clean beauty, one of the most versatile ingredients you can get your paws on. It can be used on your body, face, hair and toes. You can use it to moisturise, remove make-up, nourish hair, soothe flaky itchy skin, soften cuticles, heal insect bites and calm inflamed skin. Talk about one size fits all. If there's one thing you need to buy after reading this book, it's one bloody big jar of coconut oil.

Coconut oil is primarily comprised of medium-chain fatty acids, the saturated fats that your body loves. It means that is has a rich, solid texture and helps the skin retain its moisture content. The lauric acid in the oil also has strong antimicrobial properties, protecting the skin from infection. This benefit is also present when taken orally, as the fatty acids boost

Coco

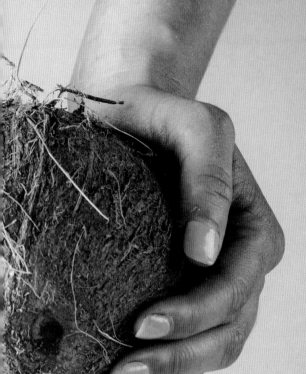

immunity when converted by the body. It is a unique substance; at room temperature it is a solid white, yet a little heat transforms it into a clear liquid.

The oil is also rich in vitamin A, which protects the degeneration of tissue, and vitamin E, a natural antioxidant. These vitamins help to prevent dehydration of the skin. We love coconut oil as an all-rounder; it can be used in hair masks, face and body scrubs, and balms. One word of advice: it is very rich, so if you have acne-prone or oily skin, best not to lather it on your face.

Some of the ways we love to use coconut oil? It makes a great base for a balm, because of it's solid and easy to work with structure. It's also great for oil pulling and you'll spot it in our Whiten Your Smile (p. 67) with activated charcoal. We've used fractionated coconut oil in a couple of recipes; this is coconut oil that has gone through steam distillation to remove the medium-chain fatty acids and keeps it from solidifying. It also extends the shelf life so it's a good addition to liquid serums that you don't want to have solid!

green with envy

1 teaspoon coconut cream
1 teaspoon spinach and/
  or kale juice (see p. 65)
1 teaspoon avocado oil

MAKES:
15ml

SHELF LIFE:
Quantities are deliberately small to ensure that the product is used within its shelf life and not wasted. Store in the fridge for up to 1 week.

HELPFUL HINT:
Can be used as a mask or eye cream, but make sure you wipe off every trace before leaving the house!

Hello, super greens! We've put together this eye cream using spinach and kale, which have become veggie superheroes in the current health craze. We're wearing our 'I Heart Kale' jumpers as we speak. As ever, what's good for your insides is also great for your outside. When you combine spinach and kale, you create a nutrient powerhouse that has been likened to natural Botox. They are rich in chlorophyll, enzymes, vitamins, minerals and phytonutrients that will leave you seriously glowing. For the delicate, fine-line-prone skin around the eyes, this is seriously good stuff. Avocado oil is rich in antioxidants but also absorbs quickly, so it is great for the eye area.

---

1 Blend the ingredients and decant into a small container.
2 Use around the eye area and wipe away any green residue before heading out.

probiotic enzyme peel

1 tablespoon lime juice
1 kiwi fruit, mashed
¼ papaya, mashed
3 tablespoons agar-agar
   jelly
1 probiotics capsule

MAKES:
One use

SHELF LIFE:
One-time use; store in the
fridge for up to 2 days.

HELPFUL HINT:
Unripe papaya contains
more of the enzyme papain,
but may cause irritation to
sensitive skin.

The notion of a peel can seem a little brutal, but we assure you, it's a great way to remove dead skin cells and show off new glowing skin. Traditionally cosmetic peels are filled with harsh synthetic acids and silicones that quite literally peel away the skin, but we've come up with a gentle natural alternative. The agar-agar jelly, found in the Japanese section of any good supermarket, is derived from seaweed and used not only as a thickening agent but also for its high mineral content of iron, magnesium and calcium. Kiwis are packed with vitamins C and E, as well as magnesium, potassium, lutein and copper. The papain enzymes in papaya gently exfoliate, evening out skin tone and removing acne-causing bacteria. The limes add an astringent quality to the mask, tightening pores and further gently exfoliating. Adding probiotics supercharges this anti-ageing peel, reducing inflammation and protecting the skin against free radicals that cause signs of ageing.

---

1 Add the lime juice to the mashed kiwi and papaya.
2 Put the agar-agar jelly in a bain-marie and stir until the jelly melts and forms a thickish paste.
3 Stir in the probiotic powder and mashed fruit when cool.
4 Place in the fridge to cool completely.
5 Apply, leaving for 15 minutes until dry, then peel off.

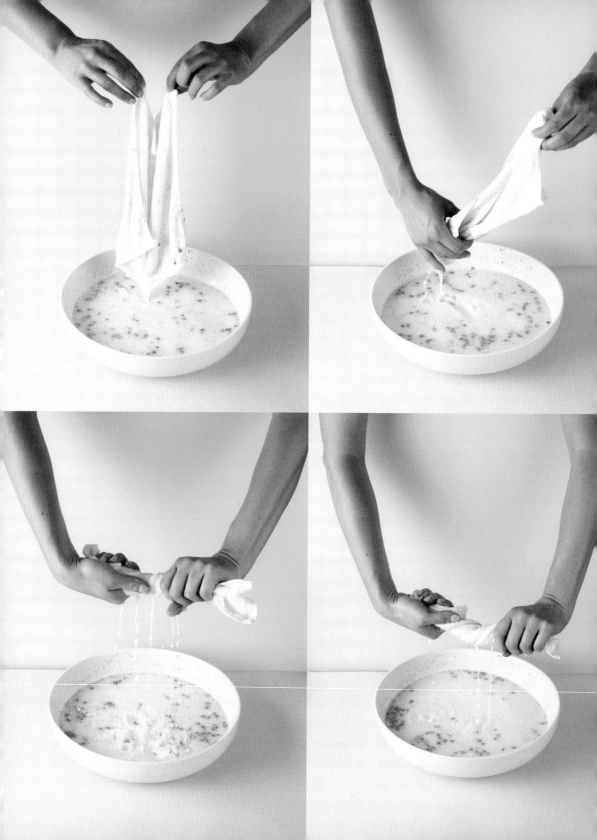

hot and steamy

½ cup chamomile tea
1 tablespoon honey
1 teaspoon grated ginger
½ cup soya milk

MAKES:
One use

SHELF LIFE:
One-time use; use
immediately.

HELPFUL HINT:
Apply a refrigerated toner
straight after the compress
to close the pores and
tighten the skin.

If you're feeling a bit grey, pressing a hot flannel soaked in this
mixture is particularly revitalising and a great pick-me-up for
skin lacking in tone. Chamomile is soothing for tired skin and
soya milk is rich in firming phytoestrogens. Ginger helps to
bring oxygen-carrying blood to the surface. Honey will ensure
skin remains soft and supple by locking in moisture. This
compress is a rich source of antioxidants; use when in need of
a glowing complexion.

1 Add the honey and ginger to the hot tea and leave for 10 minutes.
2 Stir in the soya milk.
3 Submerge a cotton flannel in the mixture and place over the face.
4 Repeat three times.
5 You can leave the residue on the skin overnight or remove
immediately.

revitalise me

50ml fennel tea, cooled

3 strawberries, mashed

2 tablespoons orange
juice

½ teaspoon honey

1 drop orange essential
oil

MAKES:
One mask

SHELF LIFE:
One-time use; use
immediately.

HELPFUL HINT:
Add your favourite
superfood powder for
an extra boost.

This is a great pick-me-up for tired, lacklustre skin that has been out for one too many margaritas (hey, no judging, we love margaritas!). Fennel tea is made from fennel seeds, which contain plant oestrogens and phytohormones that firm and rejuvenate the skin. Oranges are rich in collagen-promoting vitamin C and skin-refining acids, while the honey in this treatment is great for pepping up sluggish, mature complexions. Strawberries are a rich natural source of salicylic acid and will wipe away dead skin cells along with any unwanted traces of parties past…

1 Mix the tea with the strawberries and orange juice.
2 Blend in the honey and orange essential oil.
3 Apply to the face, rinsing off after 10 minutes.

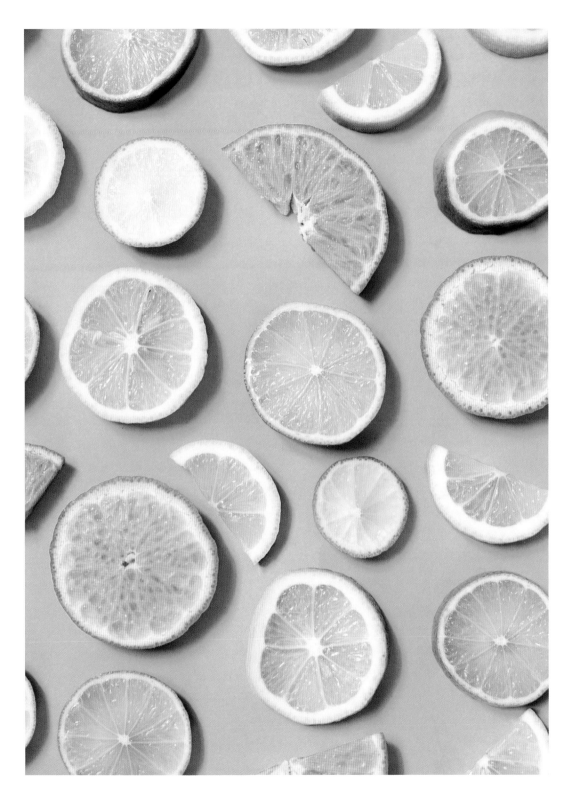

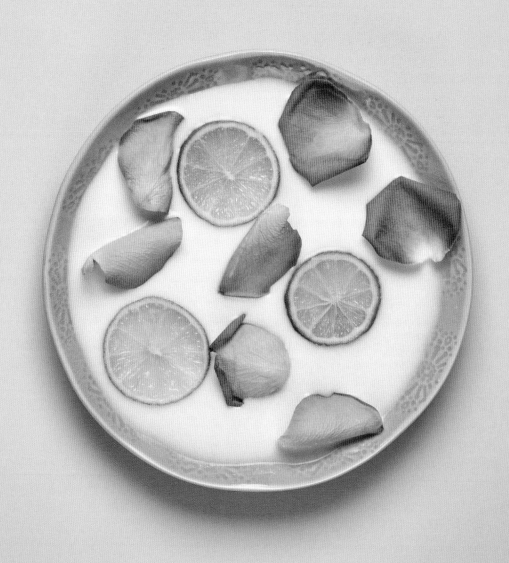

rosier glow

50ml coconut milk
50ml rosewater
1 lime, juiced

MAKES:
One soak

SHELF LIFE:
One-time use; use
immediately.

HELPFUL HINT:
You could swap the milk for
cream and make a luxurious
face mask instead.

We often soak our bodies, but tend to neglect our faces in
our bathing rituals. We don't like anyone to feel left out, so we
present to you the face bath. Slather this baby all over your
face and neck or soak a cloth and let it rest. Coconut milk
is antibacterial, antifungal and moisturising; lime is super-
rejuvenating, while rose helps to soften the skin to give you
that even rosier glow.

---

1 Gently heat the coconut milk until warm.
2 Mix all the ingredients together.
3 Leave to cool until the mixture becomes tepid.
4 Soak a cotton cloth, rest on the face and leave to soak.

mermaid mask

1 tablespoon wakame
1 tablespoon chlorella
1 tablespoon green clay
3 tablespoons water or
hydrosol
3-4 nori sheets

MAKES:
One mask

SHELF LIFE:
One-time use; use
immediately.

HELPFUL HINT:
This can get messy, so it's a
good idea to have a bowl of
clean water nearby.

Marine ingredients have been all the rage in the East for
centuries and they've finally hit our shores: nori, chlorella algae
and wakame are some of the super-healthy ingredients gracing
our plates and now we're saying let's put them on our faces!
This mask is packed with minerals and vitamins, and studies have
shown that seaweed in particular has an anti-ageing and healing
effect on the skin. Clays are naturally-occurring mineral powders
that draw impurities out of the skin, and green clay is particularly
absorbent. This one's also a double-whammy: over the mask you
place soaked sheets of nori to harness the full power of Mother
Ocean. Listen, we're going to be honest, this smells like a salty
swamp. But hold your breath and go for it, because it is SO
worth it!

---

1 Blend the wakame to a fine powder using a food processor.
2 Add the chlorella and green clay.
3 Make into a paste with water or your favourite hydrosol and apply
to the face.
4 Soak the nori sheets in water until soft.
5 Layer the sheets of nori over the face until it is completely covered.
6 When the clay has dried and the face feels tight, remove the mask
and cleanse thoroughly.

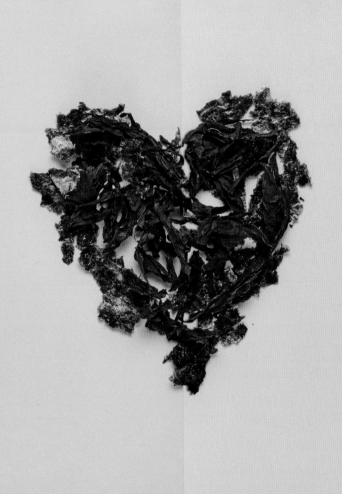

up the ante (oxidants)

A handful of blueberries
1 teaspoon yogurt
1 teaspoon chia seeds
1 capsule evening
  primrose oil

Another smoothie for the face – at least if you have leftovers, you won't go hungry! Mop up ageing free radicals and moisturise using this omega-3-rich mask. Blueberries are anti-inflammatory and protect collagen from damage, chia seeds smooth fine lines and yogurt gently wipes away dead skin cells with its lactic acid content. It's also high in probiotics: great for the stomach, great for the face.

MAKES:
One mask

SHELF LIFE:
Store in the fridge for up to 1 week.

1 In a food processor, blend the blueberries, yogurt and seeds.
2 Break the oil capsule and stir the oil into the mixture.
3 Apply to the face, washing off with a warm towel after 15 minutes.

HELPFUL HINT:
Add your favourite super-food powder for an extra boost.

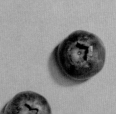

kale face rinse

A handful of kale
1 teaspoon honey

MAKES:
One rinse

SHELF LIFE:
One-time use; use
immediately.

HELPFUL HINT:
You can add spinach or
superfoods to this mix for
a nutrient power punch.

The idea behind this face rinse is to pulp the kale, extracting
the fibrous juice and then blend it with honey for a sensational
face cleanse. The nutritional composition of kale is pretty
extraordinary: rich in vitamins A, C, E and K, it is great for evening
out skin tone and tackling dark circles under the eyes. Kale is
also full of lutein, a carotenoid that helps improve skin elasticity
and hydrate the skin; kale's glucosinolates can also help regulate
detoxification. There are also 45 different flavonoids in kale,
including kaempferol and quercetin, which combine both
antioxidant and anti-inflammatory benefits. W.O.W.

1 Blend the kale in a hand blender or food processor until you see
a green liquid form.
2 Strain the mixture so you're left with the kale juice and stir the
honey into it.
3 Apply to the face as a wash, or soak a cloth and lay over the face
for 10 minutes.

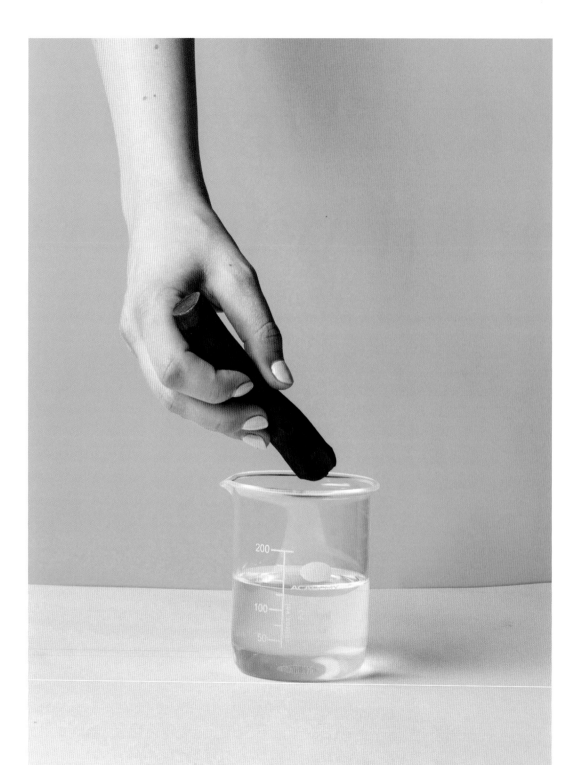

whiten your smile

1 teaspoon activated
** charcoal**
1 teaspoon coconut oil

MAKES:
One use

SHELF LIFE:
One-time use; use
immediately.

HELPFUL HINT:
The charcoal can stain
clothes so best to cover up.

Activated charcoal is one of the newest beauty discoveries and we find it particularly great for teeth whitening. No, we're not colour blind, we know it's black, which seems counterintuitive when trying to whiten, but we promise it won't leave you with a black mouth! The granules are extremely porous, pulling toxins and binding stain-causing bacteria, which will be rinsed out along with the black. Activated charcoal can also balance the pH in the mouth, and as such it's effective at preventing cavities and detoxifying the bad bacteria that cause tooth decay and gingivitis.

Activated charcoal can be found in most good health-food stores and comes either as a powder or in capsule form (just break it open to release the powder). What makes it activated, by the way, is that the charcoal has been heated to increase its absorptive properties.

---

1 Combine the activated charcoal powder and the coconut oil.
2 Dip a wet toothbrush into the charcoal and brush vigorously for at least 2 minutes.
3 Alternatively, add the charcoal powder and oil mix to a small glass of water.
4 Swirl in the mouth for 2 minutes.
5 Rinse extremely thoroughly.

I've got 99 problems
and coconut oil solved
like 86 of them.

body

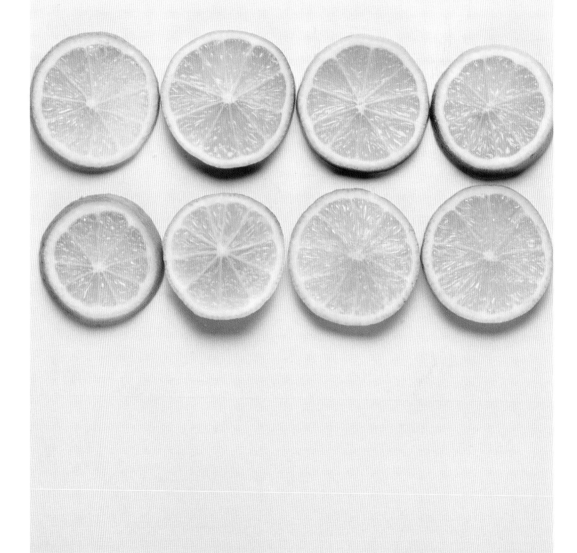

coconut cuticles

10g coconut oil
10ml olive oil
2 drops lemon essential
oil

––––––––

MAKES:
20g

SHELF LIFE:
3 months.

HELPFUL HINT:
You could put this in
an empty sterilised nail
varnish bottle for ease of
application.

We often forget about our cuticles, leaving them solely for our manicurist to attack with her little tools. The truth is, they don't need to be pushed back half as much as we think they do. They grow for a reason – to protect our nail bed – so it's important to keep them healthy and to be delicate. This recipe is super-easy to whip up and acts like a shot of nutrition for your cuticles. Coconut oil's ability to penetrate the skin quickly means that it will help soften up any dry patches in no time, and the olive oil is incredibly moisturising so will aid brittle nails, ultimately making them stronger and healthier. We add a dash of lemon as it has natural antibacterial properties and will therefore help fight any chances of the nail beds becoming infected.

––––––––

1 Melt the coconut oil in a bain-marie.
2 Add the olive oil and stir well.
3 Add the lemon essential oil.
4 Apply to the cuticles and massage into the nail beds.

mediterranean scrub

6 tablespoons used coffee grounds
2 tablespoons olive oil

MAKES:
One use

SHELF LIFE:
Use immediately or store any excess in the fridge to be used the next day.

HELPFUL HINT:
You can also go for coconut oil for a super nourishing hit, or if you're running short on time then eliminate the oil altogether and just use the coffee!

This is a great entry-level recipe for those who are keen to get involved in the coffee scrub gang but can't be bothered with a mega prepping session. It's an easy recipe that takes minutes to throw together and also benefits from being super eco-friendly as it reuses the coffee grounds that you'd usually throw away, making you a green-warrior with a super-smooth bum. We can imagine those folks in the Mediterranean just loving this combo in the morning before they go out for their daily swim in their turquoise waters because it's always sunny. Us? Jealous? No. If you've got a little more time then add some organic raw cane sugar or blitzed-up Himalayan salt for a bit more oomph on the exfoliating front.

We add a carrier oil to help bind the mixture and moisturise the skin. In this case we've gone for olive oil as it has a high essential fatty acid content, so assists the coffee in firming and smoothing stubborn areas of dry skin. Olive oil also has high amounts of Vitamin E, which is essential in both preparing and protecting the skin from everyday damage and is something that your body can't produce of its own accord so it's vital that you source it externally.

1 Scoop your used coffee grounds into a dry container, draining away any excess moisture.
2 Add the olive oil and stir well.

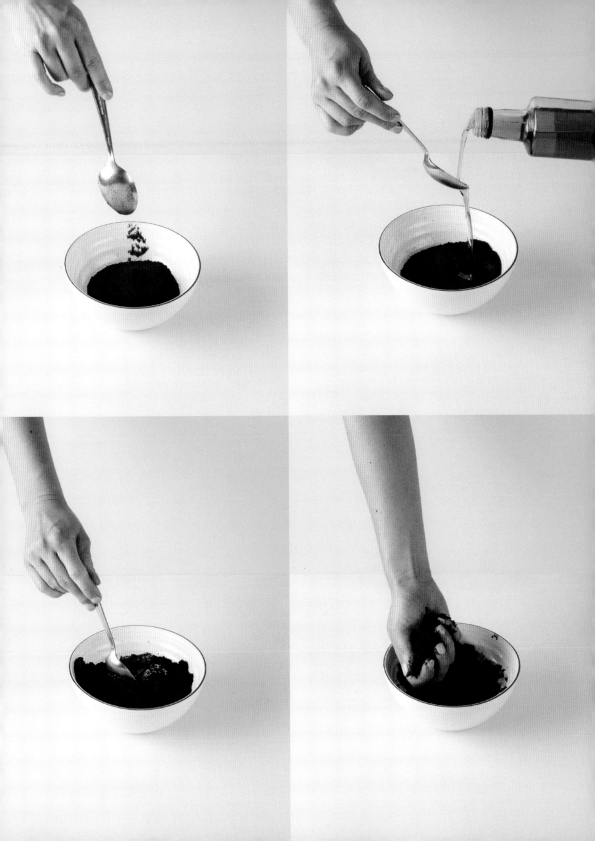

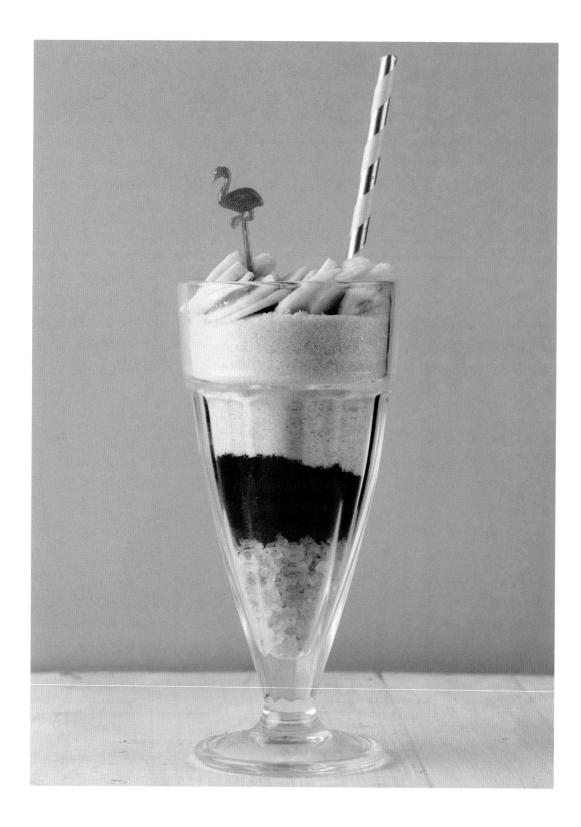

pina colada feet

1 tablespoon pink
  Himalayan salt
1 tablespoon raw cane
  sugar
1 tablespoon ground
  coffee
½ ripe banana
1 tablespoon coconut oil

MAKES:
One use

SHELF LIFE:
One-time use, store any
excess in the fridge for up
to 1 week.

HELPFUL HINT:
Coconut pulp is also an
awesome addition to this; it
adds a little extra exfoliation
and fits in with the whole
'sipping cocktails on a
hammock' vibe.

This is a bit of a magic mixture. It smells absolutely amazing and
we would 100 per cent eat it if it weren't for the salt. Resist the
urge and slather it all over your feet instead; you'll have summer-
ready trotters in no time. Skin on the feet can get especially dry
so we've gone full-on with a combo of sugar, salt and coffee as
exfoliators to shift the annoying hard skin that builds up over the
winter. We'd also recommend not blitzing the salt too much to
ensure you get a good old scrub. The potassium in the banana
and vitamin E in the coconut oil will moisturise the new skin left
behind (and leave you smelling like a tropical dreamboat).

---

1 Briefly blitz the salt in a blender to get rid of any large crystals.
2 Add the sugar and coffee and stir.
3 Add the banana and coconut oil then briefly blend again.
4 Use weekly and as you would a normal body scrub.

sweet avo body polish

½ avocado
2 tablespoons honey
½ cup oatmeal
1 tablespoon apple cider
   vinegar

MAKES:
One use

SHELF LIFE:
One-time use; use
immediately.

HELPFUL HINT:
It might seem weird
hanging around for 15
minutes covered in green
goo. We use the time to
do something handy in
the bathroom – pluck
your eyebrows, brush your
teeth, paint your toenails
– anything to pass the
time and avoid leaving the
bathroom (and risk the
danger of being seen).

We stumbled across this recipe by accident after an oatmeal
face mask got absolutely everywhere and we suddenly thought,
Hang on a minute we might be onto something here… a BODY
mask is a great idea! This is a fab combo of super-moisturising
avocado and honey with the anti-inflammatory properties of
the oats. Honey is a humectant, meaning it'll draw moisture to
your skin, so the longer you leave the mixture on, the better.
The vinegar is a really strong addition: not only is it antibacterial
and antifungal but it also unblocks pores and cleanses skin, so
it helps with any areas of acne, ingrown hairs or itchy skin across
the body. As you rinse it off, be sure to have a good scrub with
the oats – they are a great natural exfoliant!

1 Mash the avocado and mix with the honey.
2 Slowly add the oatmeal to the mixture so you have a thick paste.
3 Add the vinegar, allowing it to thin the mixture slightly.
4 Stir everything well and apply to clean, damp skin.
5 Leave for 15 minutes then rinse well.

koko kefir scrub

10g coconut oil
10g kefir yogurt
30g pink Himalayan salt

MAKES:
50g

SHELF LIFE:
1 week; store in the fridge.

HELPFUL HINT:
Leave this on for longer as a body mask if you have time. The salt will draw out impurities and balance the skin's pH.

We discovered kefir recently at CBCo. and now we're big fans. So I guess the disclaimer here is that this is a non-vegan recipe, as kefir is a dairy product. If you're down with that, read on. If not, we totally get it!

Kefir is a wonderful fermented milk, from either goats or cows, and it helps to balance the good bacteria in your gut. But as well as being awesome for your insides, it also has great benefits for the skin. It's high in alpha hydroxyl acid (AHA) which helps to regulate PH levels in the skin, ideal for areas that are feeling particularly dry or sensitive, and it is also a non-abrasive exfoliant. It has a high content of amino acids which is good to hydrate and generally nourish, plus it's actually super-easy to get hold of – you can pick up some up at any big supermarket or health food store (we've used cow kefir in this recipe as it's easier to source than goat's). We've combined it with pink Himalayan salt, which is going to remove dead skin cells, draw out impurities and remove dirt. Finally, our good friend coconut oil will provide a smooth and moisturising finish.

---

1 Melt the coconut oil in a bain-marie.
2 Allow the coconut oil to cool a little, then stir in the kefir yogurt (be careful not to let the oil solidify).
3 Add the salt to the mixture and stir into a paste.
4 Apply to a clean face and scrub away, rinsing thoroughly.

Clean beauty *and* fitness

If you're anything like us, you'll also find that you get pretty sweaty, pretty quickly (we hear it's a sign of a fast metabolism?!), and crawl out of your workout class both red-faced and drenched.

Of course you tend to jump in the shower straight away, but it's still important to ensure that your post-gym kit is going to work hard at scrubbing you up good and proper. Look out for products or recipes that are antibacterial, anti-fungal and antimicrobial. They will ensure that any bacteria left on your skin from the sweat is long gone, avoiding any infections, rashes or fungal areas so you are generally clean as a whistle. Also anything anti-inflammatory will help to relieve tired muscles!

It's a myth that exercise directly makes your skin more absorbent. It does play a part in your skin's ability to soak up what's put onto it, though, and that's why it's important to ensure your routine doesn't slip once you've been training. Here's the science bit: your skin's ability to absorb is affected by several factors, which include temperature, hydration and blood flow. Changes in all three of these things are the direct result of exercise: your skin heats up, you produce moisture to keep cool, blood circulation is increased.

So why ruin all your hard work by slathering your body with nasties when you could be providing it with nutrient-packed goodness. It's at its most absorbent after exercise so be sure to take advantage of this by developing a squeaky-clean post-gym regime. It may seem like an extra hassle to pack additional toiletries for your gym trip but it's worth the investment. Simply grab some mini containers (Boots do a good selection) and fill with your favourite natural alternatives, then keep them as your separate kit just for the gym. We love Dr Bronner's liquid soap as it's good for both face and body and provides a refreshing clean.

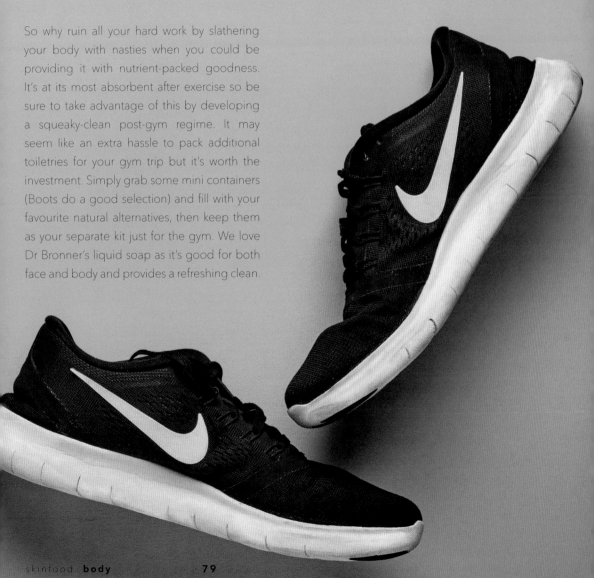

tootie-fruity tootsies

1 ripe kiwi, mashed
5 strawberries, mashed
1 tablespoon apple cider
   vinegar
1 tablespoon coconut oil

MAKES:
One use

SHELF LIFE:
One-time use; store any
excess in the fridge for up
to 3 days.

HELPFUL HINT:
The strawberries may stain
your feet a little so we
recommend you try this one
when you have a night in. If
you're desperate to remove
any stains, try a little lemon
juice.

Kiwis and strawberries are a killer combo as they are high in an array of vitamins that provide nutrients to the skin. While this may sound like a delicious smoothie (be prepared for this – it will be a recurring theme), applying topically to feet will help to hydrate, refresh, exfoliate and soften. Perfect after a long day running about town. Strawberries are incredibly high in vitamin C, which is an anti-inflammatory and helps in the healing process – so this is ideal if you have cracked or sensitive heels (no pun intended). The kiwis have tons of vitamins E and K, which help to nourish and replenish skin cells. Both are high in natural fruit acids and their little pips work as a great exfoliant. The dash of ACV is there to a) act as an antibacterial property, which helps with stinky trotters, and b) prevent you from eating the recipe before it even gets to your feet.

---

1 Combine the kiwis and strawberries and stir in the apple cider vinegar.   .
2 Add the coconut oil. This is here really to hold the mixture together so it doesn't slide off your feet.
3 Apply to feet and wrap in cling film.
4 Let sit for at least 15 minutes before rinsing off with warm water.

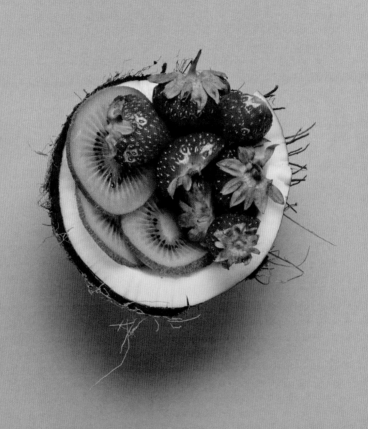

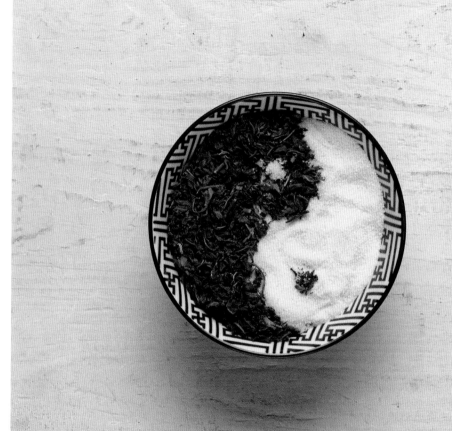

sweet tea scrub

½ cup raw cane sugar
1 tablespoon loose
   green tea
1 tablespoon honey
1 tablespoon coconut oil

_____

MAKES:
One use

SHELF LIFE:
One-time use; use
immediately.

HELPFUL HINT:
Try switching the green tea
for matcha; the antioxidant
properties will make this a
great anti-ageing scrub.

This one was inspired by a recent trip to India. Having forgotten to pack a scrub and in desperate need of exfoliating our trotters after a long day roaming the streets of Mumbai, we pulled together a makeshift concoction that actually worked out pretty well; we've used it regularly since. Luckily we don't travel anywhere without a small tub of coconut oil – we mixed this with some sugar, honey and loose green tea that we'd managed to pilfer from the hotel restaurant. Coconut oil is a great anti-inflammatory so helps to calm sore or tired skin. The sugar is a fantastic-tasting natural exfoliant and scrubs away the grime in no time. Honey is a humectant and so it attracts moisture, hydrating post-scrub skin. Finally the addition of green tea leaves you smelling magical and is a great antioxidant! Tea also has a high caffeine content, which helps to stimulate circulation and blood flow under the skin.

This is a thick, gloopy, super-sticky mixture, so be sure to rinse well! It's worth it, though: your skin will be left feeling incredibly soft and ready for a new day in India!

_____

1 Mix the sugar and tea together.
2 Add the honey and stir well.
3 Add the coconut oil – slightly melted works best – and stir again until well combined.
4 Apply to the body and start scrubbing, focusing particularly on legs and feet.

kitchen cupboard
body oil

30ml olive oil
30ml sunflower oil
20ml avocado oil
20ml almond oil

_____

MAKES:
100ml

SHELF LIFE:
6 months in an airtight container.

HELPFUL HINT:
You can add a couple of dried vanilla pods or a handful of dried flowers to the mixture to gently fragrance the oil.

The oils that we use to cook our food are often perfect for skincare too. So long as you're using high quality, organic and virgin oils, why not share the love with your shower as well as your frying pan? Many kitchen-cupboard oils are perfect for hydrating skin: they're obviously very high in fats so they provide the skin with much needed moisture. Grapeseed oil is high in beta-carotene, which the body converts to vitamin A and is essential for healthy skin. The combination we've outlined here is an absolute superstar for nourishment but it may not smell the best as we've not used anything to fragrance, so you may choose to use this as a body oil cleanser and rinse off. You'll still get the benefits of the oils but the smell won't linger as much.

_____

1 Combine all the oils and stir well.
2 Store in a pump bottle and use as and when needed.

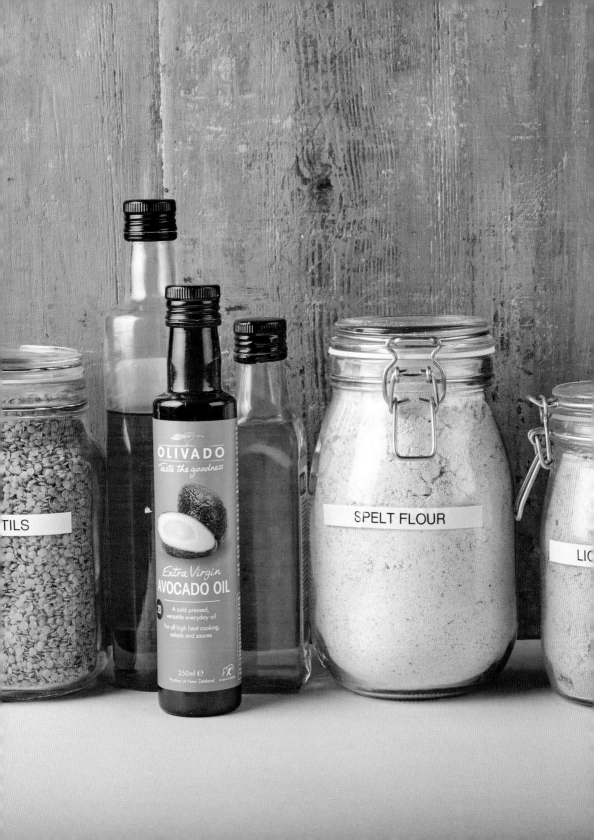

that's a wrap

**2 tablespoons rhassoul
clay**
**2 tablespoons boiled
water**
2 tablespoons olive oil
**2 tablespoons pink
Himalayan salt**
**fabric, enough for the area
to be treated**

MAKES:
One use

SHELF LIFE:
One-time use; use
immediately.

HELPFUL HINT:
You can use an old bed
sheet, muslin or bandages
or cling film (although we
prefer the former, from an
eco-friendly perspective).

This one requires a little investment as you'll need to lie in the bath, fully wrapped up like a mummy, for at least 45 minutes. So save it for one of those nights when you need a little 'me' time. When the BF's out, you have zero intention of leaving the house and there's no danger of someone strolling in mid-wrap (a terrifying experience for you both). It'll be worth it, though, trust us – this wrap will leave you feeling super smooth and will help to detox the skin and body. Ideal for pre-summer to get ready for bikini body time, or if you've generally been hitting it a little hard and the result is dry, dehydrated skin all over. We love the idea of the whole Moroccan hammam spa experience and wanted to recreate this at home, so we chose rhassoul clay as the base for this recipe, which is sourced from the Atlas Mountains (although you can get your hands on some from Amazon) and is ace at drawing out dirt, impurities and even fat from the skin. It's been used for centuries as a natural cleanser because of its ability to remove dirt gently. Salt also has absorptive properties, which will assist the clay in detoxing while also acting as an exfoliant. The high vitamin E content of olive oil will moisturise so you will honestly end up with the silkiest skin in town.

---

1 Mix the clay with the water to form a paste.
2 Meanwhile, very gently heat the olive oil until it's warm. Don't allow to boil, you just want to be working with warm oil.
3 Slowly add the oil to your clay mixture, stirring continuously, then add the salt. You should have a large quantity of a thick paste.
4 Apply the mixture to any area of your body that you'd like to treat. We generally focus on legs, bums, tums and upper arms.
5 Cover the mixture in the fabric wraps, bandaging up tightly. Relax for at least 45 minutes, to allow it to do its work.

clear as cleopatra soak

1 cup organic whole milk
2 tablespoons honey

Optional: Dried rosemary, lavender or rose petals (purely from a scent standpoint, they'll add a lovely aroma to your bath)

———————

MAKES:
One soak

SHELF LIFE:
One-time use; use immediately.

HELPFUL HINT:
You can also add Epsom salts for a super-detoxifying experience.

Let's make like the Egyptians for a second because, frankly, who doesn't want to be like Cleopatra? Luckily for us, her badass ruling isn't the only thing she's famous for today. Her beauty regime is still used by many, thousands and thousands of years later. So we're taking a leaf out the Queen's (ancient) book with her infamous recipe for soft, supple, young skin. And it's super-simple: milk and honey. That may sound like a delicious bedtime drink to you, but both ingredients have amazing benefits for the skin. Milk contains lactic acid, which is an alpha hydroxy acid (or AHA). AHA helps to regenerate skin cells faster by sloughing off dead and damaged cells. Honey is a humectant and is incredibly soothing for dry skin. So combined, the two killer ingredients will leave you with soft, rejuvenated skin and a youthful-looking glow to rival Cleo herself.

———————

1 Gently heat the milk (do not allow to boil).
2 Add the honey and stir in until fully dissolved, then take off the heat.
3 If you're using dried herbs or flowers, add them to the mixture and stir.
4 Pour the mixture into a running bath and swirl well.

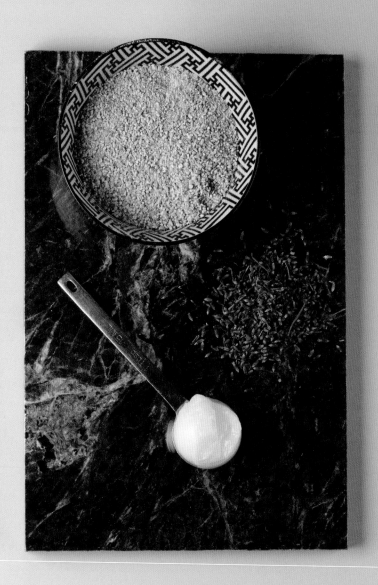

oatheal soak

90g oatmeal
10g coconut oil
5 drops lavender
   essential oil

MAKES:
100g

SHELF LIFE:
Enough for about five baths;
store in an airtight container
for up to 3 months.

HELPFUL HINT:
This may sound weird but
bear with us… If you fancy
a bit of a scrub then ditch
the grinding and keep
the oats whole. Put all the
ingredients into a pair of
tights, tie a knot in the end
and use as an exfoliant while
in the bath.

See what we did there? A funny play on oatmeal, because it really does help the skin heal. Other than making a nutritious breakfast, oats have some great benefits for the skin. They are a known anti-inflammatory so are widely used in the treatment of skin conditions such as eczema and psoriasis because they help to calm and reduce redness. They contain healthy fats that are great for moisturising the skin and also contain polysaccharides, molecules that handily become gelatinous when mixed with water and form a protective layer over the skin, which is great for hydration and soothing itchiness or irritation. We've combined the oatmeal with coconut oil, which is an ultra-gentle moisturiser and will provide nourishment without causing the skin to flare up. Finally, the addition of lavender is to help relax any discomfort of either the skin or the mind.

1 Grind the oatmeal in a blender or coffee grinder for a few minutes until it becomes extremely fine.
2 Gently heat the coconut oil in a bain-marie, add the lavender essential oil and stir well.
3 Combine the oils and oatmeal and stir.
4 Add a handful to a running bath and swirl to ensure even distribution.

triple a
(awesome antioxidant aftersun)

1 pomegranate

1 tablespoon green tea powder

2 tablespoons aloe vera gel

MAKES:
One use

SHELF LIFE:
One-time use; use immediately.

HELPFUL HINT:
Keep this in the fridge prior to use for extra cooling – all together now – ahhhhhhh.

Three ingredients, three times the antioxidant power. Unfortunately for the sun babies out there, UV rays are known to produce free radicals. Antioxidants, on the other hand, fight them. Soooo, if you've been an absolute dingbat and forgotten to apply enough sunscreen, you better be sure as hell that your aftersun packs a powerful, antioxidant punch. Enter Triple A – three ingredients that you can whip up in no time and will immediately get to work on your damaged and tender skin. Both pomegranate and green tea are incredibly high in antioxidants and are known to combat skin damage and help fight signs of ageing. Combined, they'll combat the harm that those free radicals will be causing. Aloe has been used for centuries on burns as it has high antibacterial and anti-inflammatory properties that immediately soothe and fight further infection. And the best part? Aloe is also a powerful antioxidant. The three together will help remedy your sunscreen blunder. Just don't make a habit of it.

---

1 Scoop out the fleshy insides from the pomegranate and blend into a pulp.

2 Add the green tea and stir well.

3 Add the aloe vera gel and blend again until you have a smooth paste.

4 Apply to affected areas and allow to sit for as long as you can.

5 It's very sticky so you'll need to wash it off eventually but the longer you can leave it on, the better.

oil and vinegar cellulite buster

20ml olive oil
10ml apple cider vinegar

MAKES:
30ml

SHELF LIFE:
3 months in an airtight container.

HELPFUL HINT:
Add a drop of grapefruit essential oil for the ultimate cellulite buster.

Apple cider vinegar really is great. It's fantastic when consumed: it helps with weight loss and gut health, is high in folic acid and vitamins B1, B2 and C, and is incredibly antibacterial. But we like to use it topically on the skin as (you guessed it) many of these benefits help keep your outside just as healthy as your inside. This particular recipe is aimed at cellulite because ACV is often linked to speeding up metabolic rate and helping with blood flow. The molecules of the vinegar stimulate circulation and have what is almost a melting effect on areas of high fat build-up and cellulite. Obviously there are many causes of cellulite and both diet and exercise will contribute to helping reduce it, but this will help to smooth out the skin in the surrounding areas and improve general appearance. The addition of olive oil allows it to glide on smoothly and helps the ACV to penetrate the top layer of the skin.

---

1 Mix the olive oil and vinegar together.
2 The two will naturally separate so you'll need to shake well before use. Massage onto dry skin on all areas affected by cellulite. Leave for up to 10 minutes before rinsing off thoroughly.

Why is it called beauty
sleep when you wake up
looking like a troll?

hair

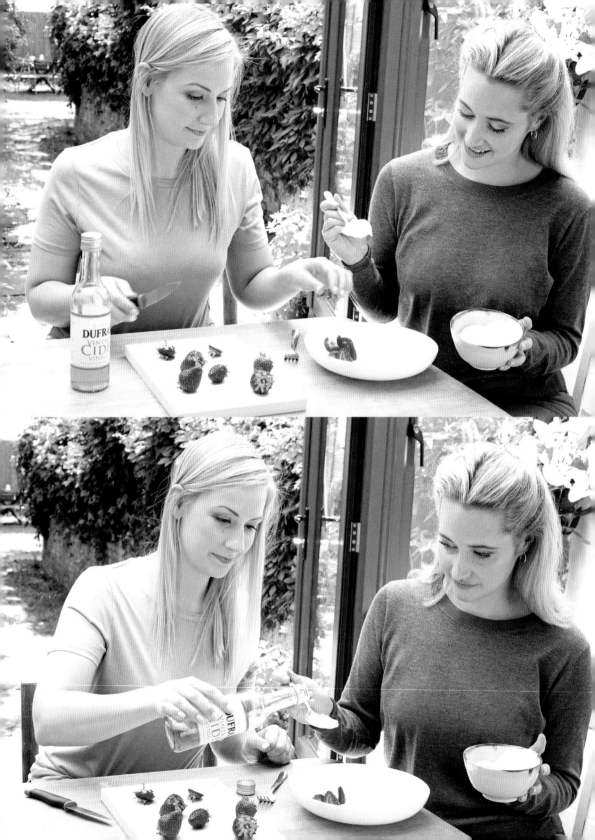

berry good hair

2 tablespoons natural
   yogurt
3 strawberries, mashed
2 tablespoons apple cider
   vinegar

MAKES:
One mask

SHELF LIFE:
One-time use; any leftovers
can be stored in the fridge
for up to 1 week.

HELPFUL HINT:
For an extra moisture kick,
add a dash of honey!

Can strawberries do no wrong? They are such superstars in providing the ultimate nutrients while also being just so tasty. We like them for our hair because they contain high levels of silica, which has been linked to preventing hair loss. At the risk of sounding like we're making a delicious breakfast pot, we've also added yogurt because it is extremely high in protein, which is essential for strong hair. On top of that it's got a high lactic acid content, which acts as a great exfoliant, gently clearing away dead skin cells at the scalp, which, combined with the ACV, makes for healthy hair at the roots. All in all, it's a simple yet effective treatment for instant lustrous locks.

1 Combine the yogurt and strawberries.
2 Add the apple cider vinegar and stir well.
3 Push the mixture through a sieve to remove the pithy bits of strawberry.
4 Apply the paste to wet hair, covering from root to tip, and allow to sit for up to 30 minutes.
5 Rinse well and shampoo twice to ensure the hair is totally clean.

camu camu swim spray

3g camu camu powder
35ml boiling water
2g bicarbonate of soda
10ml aloe vera gel

_____

MAKES:
50ml

SHELF LIFE:
Up to 1 week in the fridge
without a preservative;
3 months with.

HELPFUL HINT:
We also use this before we
get in the pool as we find
that the aloe provides a
protective layer over the hair.

This recipe came about after the pair of us took on an Olympic-distance triathlon (absolute nutters) and were constantly in the pool trying to get our swimming skills up to scratch for the epic 1.5km distance. We really noticed the effect that the chlorine had on our hair, particularly as we're both blonde. We were often left with dry, tangled and unmanageable hair that stank of chlorine. Not attractive in any way. We did a bit of research and discovered that vitamin C works a treat, neutralising the harsh effects that the chemical has. Camu camu is an Amazonian fruit that has one of the highest vitamin C levels of any natural plant: perfect for pumping nutrients back into chlorine-frazzled hair. It's widely available in powder form, so we've combined it with cooling and soothing aloe that'll mix perfectly in water to develop a handy little spray. Finally, vitamin C has a pretty acidic pH level, which may cause scalp sensitivities. We've popped in a bit of bicarb, which is extremely alkaline and will balance out the pH of the entire mixture, as well as evening out any green tones on blondes.

_____

1 Dissolve the camu camu powder in the boiling water and stir well.
2 Add the bicarbonate of soda and aloe and stir again until everything has dissolved.
3 Decant into a spray bottle and spritz over clean wet hair. Dry and style as normal.

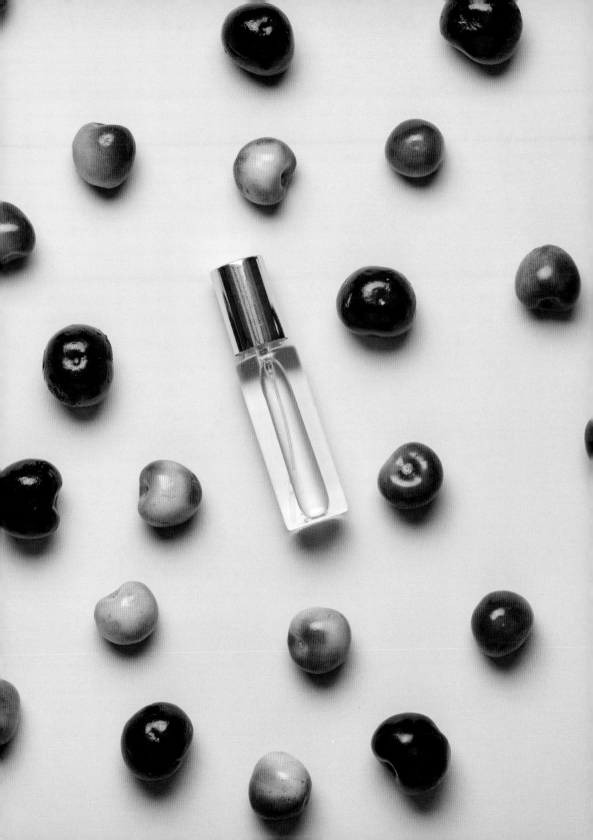

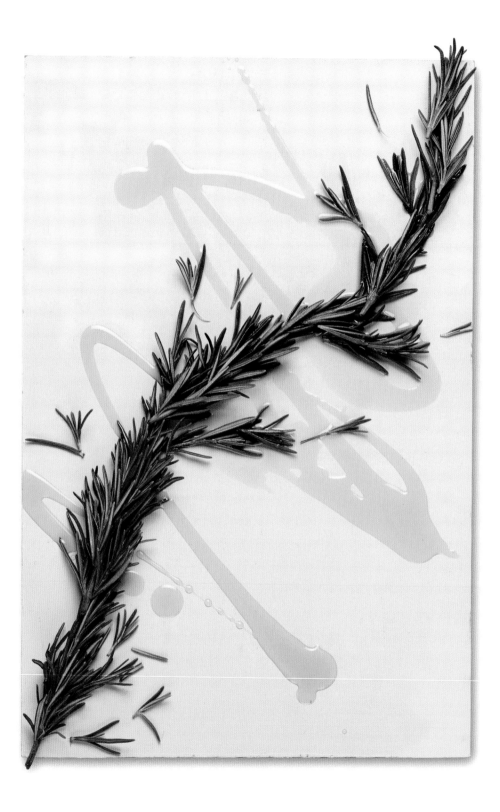

rosemary grow

3 tablespoons olive oil
A handful of dried
rosemary sprigs

MAKES:
One treatment

SHELF LIFE:
3 months in an airtight
container.

HELPFUL HINT:
If you find olive oil too heavy,
replace with grapeseed oil.

The combo of rosemary and olive oil may sound like an accompaniment to roast chicken, but it's actually a fab little treatment to help encourage hair growth. There are many factors that play into hair loss and the rate your hair grows and we're not here to solve them all. Instead, what this recipe does is strive for a healthy scalp, ensuring it's in the best possible condition when it comes to new hair growth. Rosemary is the perfect herb to do this: it's got strong antibacterial and cleansing properties that help to unclog any blocked pores on the scalp, ensuring the hairs can grow. It's also a powerful herb in its ability to stimulate circulation and blood flow, in turn aiding the production of new hair.

---

1 Gently heat the olive oil in a bain-marie.
2 Add the rosemary and cover the pan.
3 Allow to simmer on a very low heat for a couple of hours, making sure the pan of water doesn't boil dry.
4 Remove from the heat and allow to cool.
5 Strain through a sieve to remove all the rosemary and store in an airtight bottle.
6 Apply a teaspoonful to the ends of clean, wet hair, leave for 30 minutes and rinse thoroughly, shampooing as normal.

volume spritz

½ cup boiling water
1 teaspoon coconut oil
1 teaspoon pink
   Himalayan salt
1 teaspoon aloe vera gel

MAKES:
50ml

SHELF LIFE:
2–3 weeks in the fridge.
Add a broad-spectrum
preservative (see p. 212) and
it can last up to 6 months.

HELPFUL HINT:
Keep in the fridge for an
ultra-refreshing spritz! This
one will cool down the
hottest of heads in no time.

With this spritz we're trying to create the voluminous and effortless manes we tend to sport on holidays. The salt in the mixture sticks to your hair fibre to create that choppy, loose wave effect that's an essential part of the bed-head look. Salt, however, is absorbent so you do run the risk of moisture being sucked from the hair follicles. To counteract this, we've included our trusty coconut oil to keep your locks smooth and silky. We've also popped in a bit of aloe vera, which again will ensure moisture levels stay strong, and will also act as a hair gel, keeping your newly-found beach waves intact. Give this a whirl if you want to look less beach bum and more beach babe.

----

1 Bring the water to the boil and add the coconut oil and salt. Stir well until both have dissolved.
2 Crush the kelp extract and add to the mixture, again stirring until totally dissolved.
3 Decant into a spray bottle and shake well before use, as the coconut oil will separate from the rest of the mixture.

apple cider vinegar rinse

50ml apple cider vinegar
150ml boiling water

MAKES:
One use

SHELF LIFE:
One-time use; use
immediately.

HELPFUL HINT:
It's not recommended to
use this more than once
fortnightly if you're heading
out into the sun or if you
have dyed dark hair, as it
can make the hair brittle
over time.

Sit down for this one: it might come as a bit of a shock but apple cider vinegar is actually one of your DIY staples. Its acidity helps to balance pH levels, as well as improving the hair's porosity, meaning it'll be able to absorb more moisture. It's incredibly antibacterial, thus blocking clogged follicles and promoting hair growth at the root, and has strong antifungal properties that help eliminate infection and conditions like dandruff. From a vanity point of view, ACV flattens the hair shaft, which creates a smooth finish where light will more naturally bounce off. The result of this is a shiny mane that'll give even Jennifer Aniston a run for her money. Super-simple to use, it's a total superstar ingredient. This one's great to use after a few of our shampoo recipes that raise the pH of the scalp.

---

1 Combine the ACV and water in a large jar or jug and allow to cool.
2 After shampooing and conditioning, pour the entire mixture over the hair, from root to tip.
3 Rinse well and dry as usual.

banana head

½ ripe banana
1 tablespoon olive oil
1 tablespoon honey

MAKES:
One mask

SHELF LIFE:
One-time use; use
immediately.

HELPFUL HINT:
Blitzing the banana is
important – if it has any
lumps they'll stick to your
hair and be tough to wash
out!

We go bananas for bananas at CBCo. They're a fab skin food
ingredient: nutrient-rich and with the perfect texture to provide
a base for luxurious masks. Your hair will love bananas as they
are high in potassium and vitamin B, both great for injecting
some life into dry hair. Potassium has also been linked to hair
growth. When combined with the high fat content of olive oil
and the humectant properties of honey, you basically have a
strong contender for any store-bought hair mask, just without
the synthetic ingredients.

---

1 Blitz the banana in a food processor until it's completely puréed.
2 Add the olive oil and honey, stirring well.
3 Apply to wet, combed hair. Once all the mixture has been
applied, comb through your hair again and leave to sit for up to
30 minutes. Rinse well, shampoo and condition as normal.

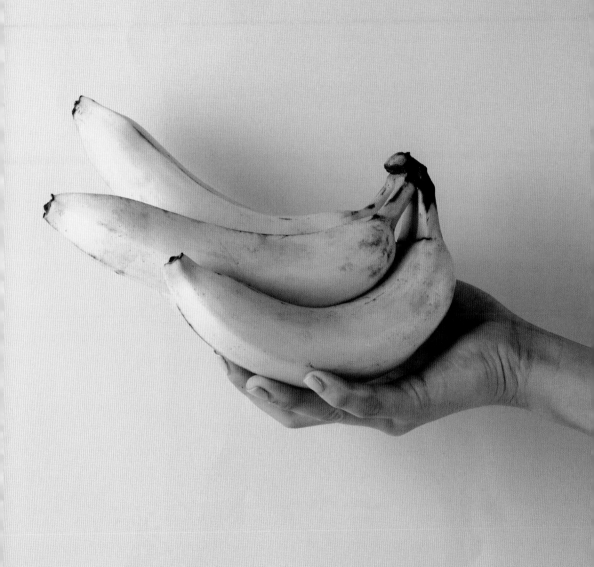

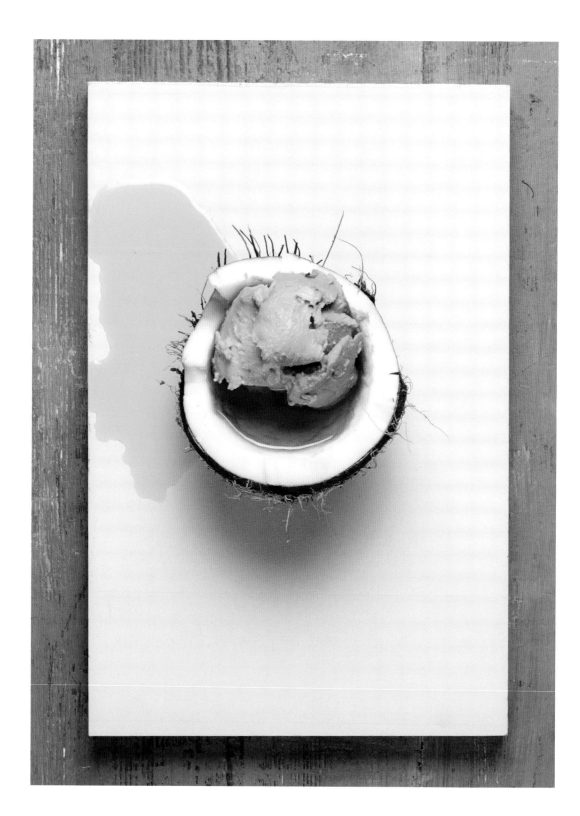

avo coco mask

2 tablespoons coconut oil
½ ripe avocado, mashed

MAKES:
One mask

SHELF LIFE:
One-time use. Leftovers can
be stored in the fridge for
up to 3 days.

HELPFUL HINT:
This is great for dandruff
or sore scalps as it's so
moisturising, so be sure to
massage well into the scalp.

Now we know exactly what you're going to say: you can't possibly use one of your beloved avos on anything other than toast, because that's what they're made for, right? Just hear us out on this one; we promise your hair will love you. Avocados are a good source of proteins and amino acids – both of which will nourish hair while promoting a healthy and moisturised scalp. Our old favourite coconut oil is an absolute babe when it comes to your hair. Its molecular structure actually means that it's able to penetrate the hair shaft much faster than other oils, conditioning from within and plumping the strand. It also reduces the loss of proteins, resulting in healthier hair and all the shine that comes with it. And the best thing about this one…? You can eat the other half of the avo on toast while you wait for the mask to set.

---

1 Melt the coconut oil in a bain-marie.
2 Combine with the avocado.
3 Apply to dry hair, covering from root to tip.
4 Allow to sit for up to 30 minutes and rinse well.

Manuka me,

When looking to buy honey for beauty reasons (or indeed to eat it) pay attention to what it's called on the label.

We've souped up a ton of recipes in the book using honey: it's a humectant which means it draws moisture in and retains it, making it perfect for healing and protecting dry skin. It blends with oils and butters, as well as working in one-time use face and hair masks. Because of its high sugar content, it's also self-preserving, so has a long shelf life and is safe to use. Though remember, if you introduce water, you need to add a preservative!

That silky golden supermarket honey is practically devoid of any nutrients or beneficial properties as it's been heated and processed to within an inch of its life. As we all know, words like 'pure' and 'natural' have no legal definitions. You're aiming for raw honey, organic honey or, better yet, organic raw Manuka honey. Manuka originates from New Zealand and it is this honey that is abundant in antibacterial and antifungal qualities. It contains vitamins, minerals and antioxidants, including calcium, iron, magnesium, sodium, zinc and vitamin C. Spot treatment? Tick! Healing scars? Tick! Skin sensitivity? Tick! Most brands rate their Manuka by its strength, and you're after a 12+ if you want to see a difference when applying it topically. Winning!

P.S You'll see we've just called honey 'honey' in our recipes; we're leaving it up to you to source the best quality you can find – raw, raw and organic, Manuka, organic Manuka is the order of the wishlist.

Manuka me not?

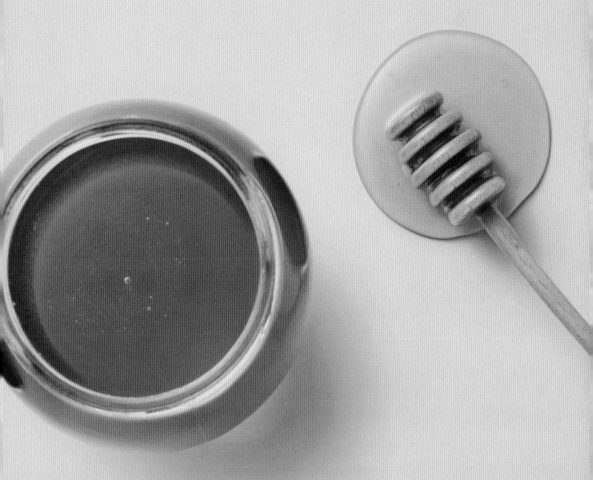

blonde ambition

½ cup chamomile tea
1 lemon, juiced
1 tablespoon honey
½ large potato, peeled
   and grated

MAKES:
One mask

SHELF LIFE:
One-time use; use
immediately.

HELPFUL HINT:
You can even blast a
hairdryer over your head
for a couple of minutes to
accelerate the lightening!

Call us biased, but we definitely believe that blondes have more fun. What is NOT fun, however, is beautiful blondies transforming into that grim brassy colour once the highlights start to fade. Golden locks quickly turn yellow without a bit of attention. There are tons of high-street brands that do the silver shampoos aimed at adding ashy tones to hair. We've come up with a natural alternative that harnesses the power of chamomile and the way its natural pigment works with blonde hair. It brings out the silvery tones of the hair, masking any red undertones, so the result is ashy goodness! We added lemon as it has natural lightening qualities, particularly if you head out into the sun. The acidity in the lemon also helps to break down the enzymes of the potato and together they have a whitening and brightening effect on blonde locks. Potatoes are rich in vitamin C, niacin, iron and zinc – nutrients that your hair loves, particularly dyed locks. The lemon can sometimes be harsh on drier hair, so we've popped in honey to moisturise and soothe.

1 Brew the tea: you want this fairly concentrated so it's fine to use a whole bag in half a cup of boiled water and allow it to steep for a while.
2 Stir both the lemon and the honey into the tea, dissolving the honey.
3 Add the potato to the mix and stir until you have a paste.
4 Apply this mixture to clean, wet hair. Massage from root to tip.
5 Wrap your head in an old towel (that you don't mind getting a little grubby) or a shower cap.
6 Allow to sit for up to 20 minutes.
7 Rinse, shampoo and condition as normal.

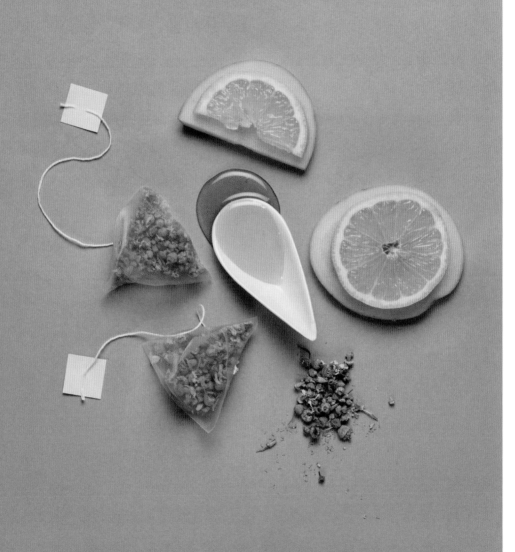

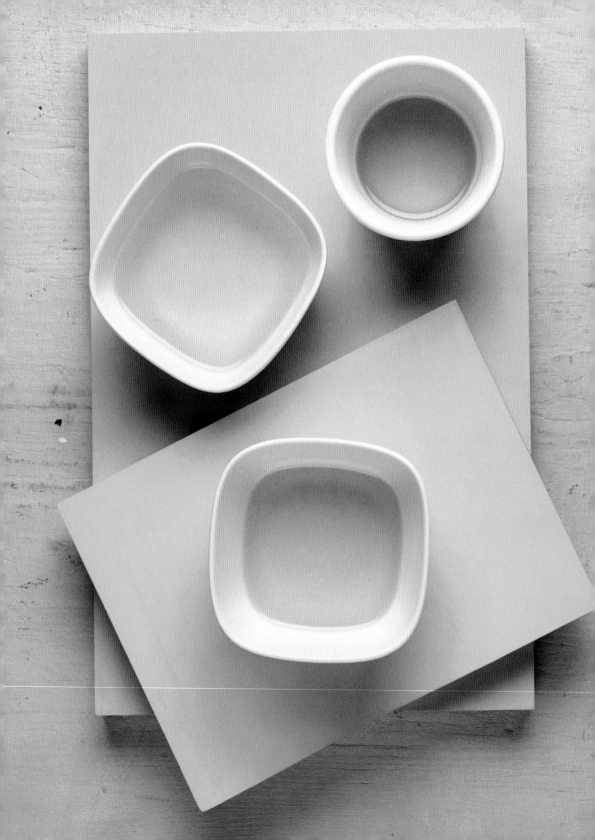

hot oil miracle treatment

1 tablespoon coconut oil
1 tablespoon olive oil
1 tablespoon avocado oil

MAKES:
One treatment

SHELF LIFE:
You could make a larger batch and keep for up to 6 months in an airtight container.

HELPFUL HINT:
It's a rich treatment so for thin or oily manes, it's best to avoid the roots and just apply to the lengths.

This one packs quite a punch, yet it's made from three very simple kitchen oils. All three are packed full of protein, which is essential for healthy hair growth and condition. They are also high in vitamin E, which your body doesn't produce naturally, so must be sourced externally. This keeps the scalp strong yet supple and encourages cell renewal, in turn promoting hair growth. The oils not only coat the outside layer of the hair, creating a shiny and glossy finish, but they're also able to penetrate the follicle, meaning hair is plumped. The beauty of this one is the process of heating – the heat helps to open the hair follicles, allowing the oils to penetrate deeper.

---

1 Melt the coconut oil in a bain-marie.
2 Combine with the other oils and leave to heat gently for a few minutes.
3 Leave to cool slightly, you want a warm mixture that isn't too hot to touch.
4 Apply to wet hair, focusing on the tips.
5 Wrap your head in a hot towel to retain the heat and leave it on for up to 1 hour.
6 Rinse thoroughly, shampoo twice and dry and style as normal.

melt away bad hair days

3 tablespoons coconut oil
2 tablespoons aloe vera
1 tablespoon honey

MAKES:
5 melts

SHELF LIFE:
You could freeze these and use as required, they will last up to 6 months in the freezer.

HELPFUL HINT:
If your hair is particularly dry, allow to sit for a few hours if possible.

These are nifty little melts that take a bit of prep, but once they're done you'll have them ready to use as and when you need them. Aloe is an overlooked ingredient in haircare; its ability to soothe, combined with its strong antibacterial and antioxidant properties, makes for a great regenerative ingredient for the scalp. Honey and its antimicrobial properties assist in cleansing the scalp of toxins and impurities that could lead to hair loss. We've spoken about the benefits of coconut oil and hair; it's an absolute superstar. In this case its strong antifungal properties will help keep the hair and scalp clean and functioning well. These melts smell lovely and are great, whether you need an extra nourishment boost or an intense conditioning treatment.

---

1 With an electric whisk, blend all the ingredients together until smooth. Your coconut oil may melt a little in the process; this is fine.
2 Scoop the mixture into a regular ice-cube tray and place in the freezer for a few hours.
3 Store in the fridge and use as and when needed. To use, apply one melt to wet hair and massage into scalp. Allow to sit for up to 5 minutes, then rinse and shampoo as normal.

coco loco detangler

½ cup coconut oil
½ cup organic coconut
    milk

MAKES:
One use

SHELF LIFE:
One-time use; use
immediately.

HELPFUL HINT:
Use as an overnight
treatment if you have
super-dry hair.

Coconut milk is a great conditioning treatment as it has many of the same properties of the oil, with the added benefit of being super-high in protein and saturated fats that nourish and moisturise dry and split ends. The combination of milk and oil in this recipe makes for an incredibly rich conditioning balm that'll detangle even the most matted of manes, coating each strand and acting as a lubricant to separate and allow combs to glide through. This is great for parched locks: post holiday, festival or if you swim a lot, as it'll moisturise and help hair become much more manageable.

---

1 Melt the coconut oil in a bain-marie.
2 Take off the heat and slowly add the coconut milk, stirring constantly.
3 Once combined, decant into a jar and allow to cool in the fridge.
4 To use, apply to the ends of wet hair after shampooing.
5 Thoroughly comb through, then rinse well.
6 You may need to shampoo again to make sure the mixture is rinsed out completely.

choco locks

2 tablespoons coconut oil
2 tablespoons honey
2 tablespoons apple cider
  vinegar
2 tablespoons cacao
  powder

MAKES:
One use

SHELF LIFE:
One-time use; use
immediately.

HELPFUL HINT:
If you have particularly
greasy hair, you can leave
out the coconut oil and just
dilute the ACV with an equal
amount of boiled water.

Cacao has a great natural pigment, so if you want to give your brunette hair a bit of a colour boost, it's a nice ingredient to include in a mask. Mixing it with an acidic ingredient like apple cider vinegar allows the colour to penetrate the hair follicles, and of course you get the benefit of the shine and lustre that the ACV brings. Honey and coconut oil are both incredibly nutritious for the hair and the latter is also antibacterial, so it will give your mane a bit of a clean while it's there.

---

1 Melt the coconut oil in a bain-marie.
2 Stir in the honey and ACV.
3 Add the cacao to the mixture last, stirring continuously to ensure there are no lumps.
4 Massage into the hair from root to tip. Allow to sit for up to 10 minutes.
5 Rinse, shampoo and condition as normal.

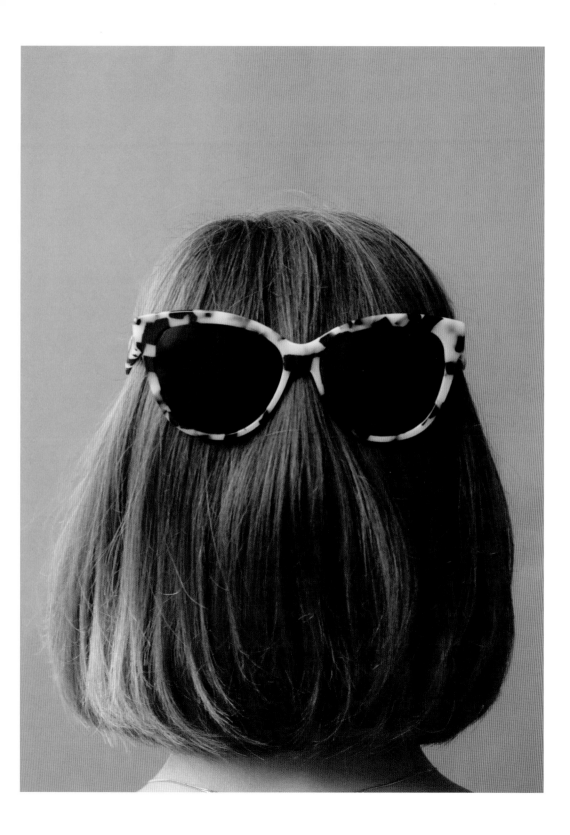

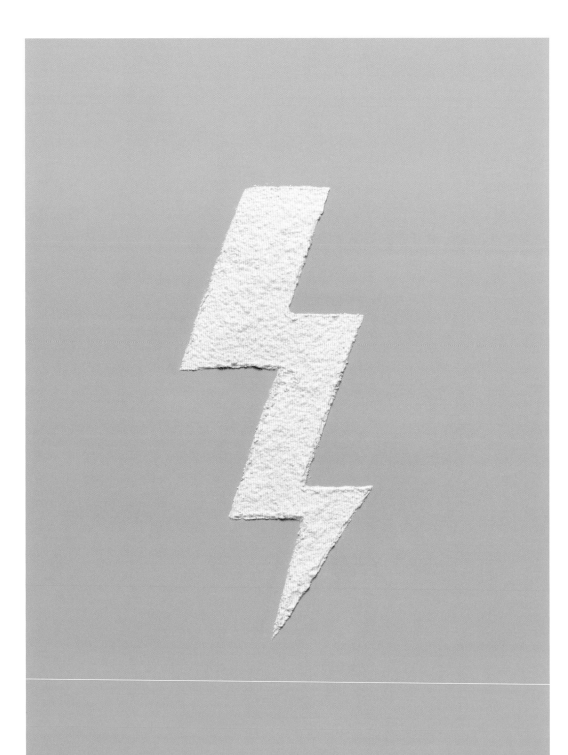

grease lightning

45g cornmeal
5g bicarbonate of soda

MAKES:
50g

SHELF LIFE:
3 months in an airtight container.

HELPFUL HINT:
If you have darker hair you may find this too light. Add a teaspoon of cocoa to darken the mixture.

We were absolute Batiste dry shampoo converts for a long time. It's so handy having a little pocket full of fresh hair goodness, despite the fact you haven't washed it for days. This is a quick-fix alternative, minus the slightly overpowering cherry scent. Head to the 'DIY Beauty: Hair' section for the full recipe (Lazy Girls' Shampoo, p.187), but this is fab to keep in the bathroom for those emergencies when you don't have anything ready and have woken up too late to wash your hair. Plus it's so easy to make. We suggest storing it in a salt or pepper shaker so that it's on hand when you need it. The cornmeal is super-porous, so it absorbs the grease and dirt at the root of the hair. The bicarbonate of soda is a nice touch as it's antibacterial and helps to clean up that greasy mop.

---

1 Combine both ingredients and stir.
2 Transfer to a salt or pepper shaker and apply to roots when needed.

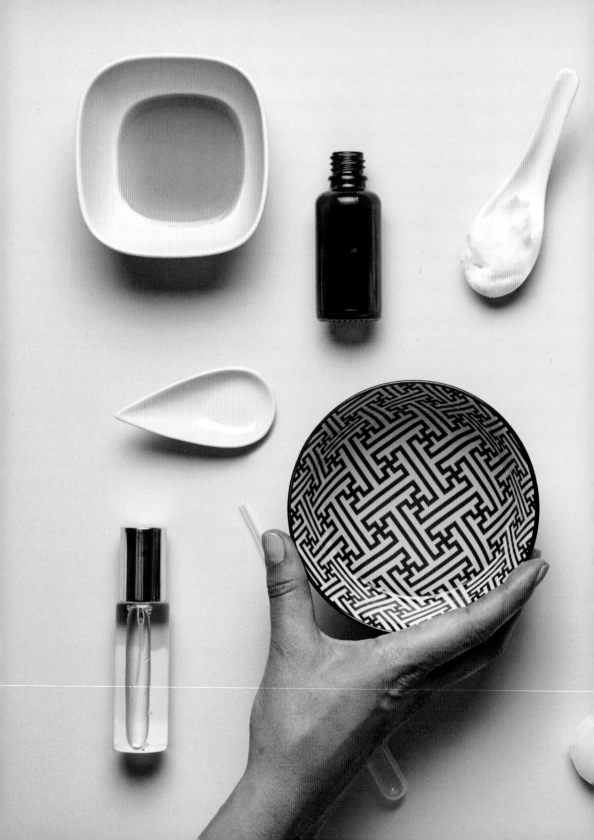

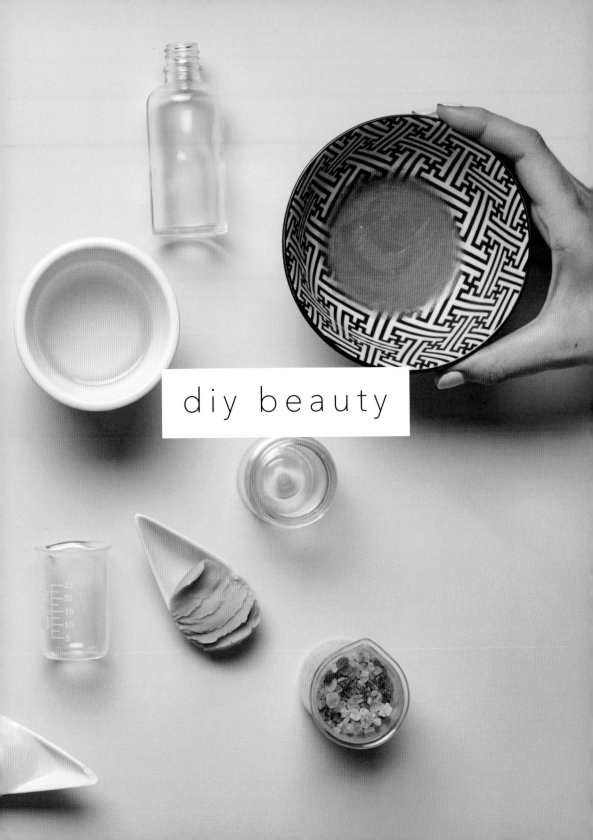

diy beauty

Looking to throw together your very own, super-moisturising, anti-ageing, gravity-defying face serum? Here are our best DIY recipes. Involving ingredients you might not have lying around, these recipes are for delving deeper into the world of Clean Beauty. Go on, give it a try. We dare you...

face

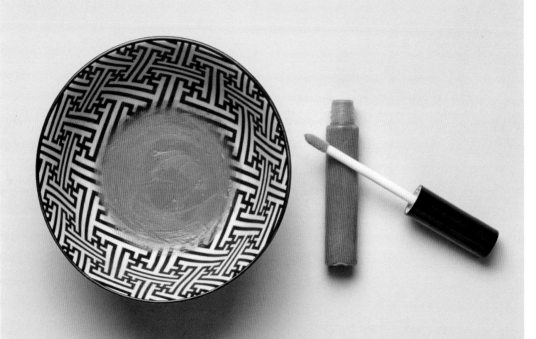

hopeless romantic gloss

3g beeswax
3g shea butter
3ml castor oil
1g pink mica

MAKES:
10ml

SHELF LIFE:
6 months in an airtight container; less if you use your fingers to apply it!

HELPFUL HINT:
Get creative with packaging; you could try a traditional lip gloss tube or the squeezy variety.

Time to pucker up! Castor oil is thick and glossy, so it's a perfect addition to the traditional butter and wax base of natural lip products. Many mainstream brands use a questionable blend of synthetic colourants and lead in lipsticks and glosses that all sit a bit dangerously close to our mouth. Mica is a natural colourant, 100 per cent non-irradiated mineral powder that has a slightly pearly undertone. It comes in many shades, and the strong raspberry pink is our favourite for a fruity lip gloss. You can flavour this with an essential oil or leave it plain.

---

1 Melt the beeswax and shea butter in a bain-marie.
2 Gently blend in the castor oil and mica.
3 This mixture cools very quickly so transfer to your container immediately.
4 If it solidifies, you can re-melt it in the bain-marie.

tropical bliss lips

6g beeswax
6g shea butter
6g mango butter
11ml apricot kernel oil
1 drop vitamin E oil

———————

MAKES:
30g

SHELF LIFE:
6 months in an airtight
container. Only apply with
clean hands.

HELPFUL HINT:
You can use candelilla wax
if seeking a vegan alternative
to beeswax.

Beeswax is included in most lip products as it leaves a layer on the lips to protect against the elements: great for dry skin and chapped lips. Soothing and softening mango butter has wonderful emollient properties and apricot oil is moisturising and regenerative. This recipe is easy to customise, so do experiment with different butters and oils; just maintain the ratios of wax, butter and oil. We love this combo of mango and apricot as it reminds us of a tropical beach… Where are our pina coladas?

———————

1 Melt the wax and butters together in a bain-marie.
2 Blend in the oil and vitamin E.
3 Decant into a lip balm tube or pot.
4 This mixture solidifies quickly so re-melt in the bain-marie if it solidifies before you've managed to decant it into your container.

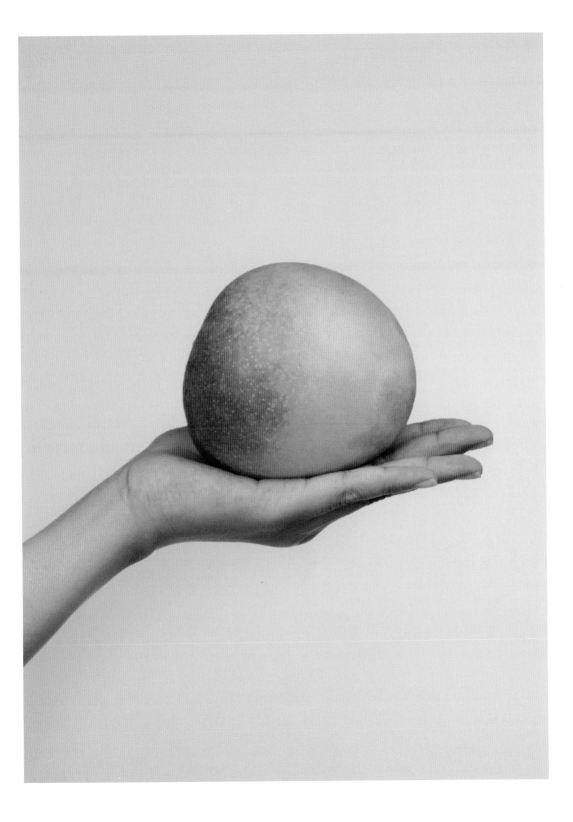

be my valentine

5g dried rose petal powder
5g raw organic cacao powder
3g rose or pink clay powder
15ml rose hydrosol

MAKES:
One mask

SHELF LIFE:
The powders will sit in an airtight container for up to 3 months. Clays are incredibly difficult to preserve naturally, so it's best to add the hydrosol only at the point of use.

HELPFUL HINT:
Spot the difference between cacao and cocoa; the latter is the slightly nutrient-inferior sibling that has been roasted at high temperatures. Sadly this destroys many of the enzymes and nutrients that make this superfood great.

Who doesn't love chocolate? We try to veer away from eating it too often (as if that ever works!) but lucky for us, it turns out it's great for your skin. We absolutely heart this chocolate and rose face mask, and if a slither lands in your mouth instead of around it, we're saying it doesn't count because accidents happen. Cacao and rose are a slick power couple, the Jay and Bey of the beauty world. Cacao is a tasty chocolate powder, rich in minerals like calcium, potassium and zinc; it's packed with antioxidants, and contains anti-inflammatory properties. The compounds found in cacao are found in plants that promote healthy skin tissue. The roses – powder, clay and hydrosol – are toning and regenerative. They help mature skin, firming and detoxifying, as well as aiding in relaxing the mind and being intoxicating to the senses. Pink clay is also a wonderfully soothing mineral powder, while at the same time drawing out impurities from the skin.

---

1 Mix the powders together slowly with the hydrosol to make into a thick paste.
2 Apply all over the face and neck and remove after 15 minutes.
3 If the clay becomes dry, pat with water to rehydrate.

eliminating serum

20ml jojoba oil
20ml rosehip oil
5ml tamanu oil
4ml sea buckthorn oil
2 drops vitamin E oil

MAKES:
50ml

SHELF LIFE:
6 months in an airtight
container.

HELPFUL HINT:
Keep serums in sterilised,
dark bottles to slow
down the oxidation and
preserve the potency of the
ingredients.

Scars affect us all, carried (literally and figuratively) in some way from mistakes we make in our youth: a heavy-handed upper-lip wax, aggressive zit popping and drunken stumbles to name a few. Rosehip and sea buckthorn do wonders for cell renewal: they are rich in omega-7 and other essential fatty acids that promote frequent cell turnover. However, the new star on the block is tamanu. The oil, extracted from the kernels of the Polynesian tamanu tree, has the ability to promote the formation of new tissue and in turn the growth of healthy skin. Its gentle composition has made it naturally hypoallergenic, and perfect for treating many sensitive skin conditions such as eczema and dermatitis. These super oils pack a punch!

---

1 Blend all the oils together.
2 Add the vitamin E.
3 Decant into a dark pump bottle.

micellar water

5ml rosehip oil
5ml castor oil
1 drop vitamin E oil
90ml rosewater

MAKES:
30ml

SHELF LIFE:
3 months if using pre-
preserved rosewater;
1 week, if not.

HELPFUL HINT:
Store in the fridge for an
extra cooling sensation
when applied.

Micellar water has become pretty trendy recently – just about every beauty brand on the block is making one. It's a magical one-stop cleanser, moisturiser and make-up remover. Maybe we're all getting lazier or maybe we just don't have enough time to go through a sophisticated three-step skincare routine twice a day. Either way, the water is something of a busy-girl's treasure, and we've put together a super simple and effective clean beauty version. The ingredients remove impurities from the skin, tone and moisturise, all in one fell swoop!

---

1 Blend the oils and vitamin E, and stir into the rosewater.
2 The oil and water will separate, so be sure to shake vigorously before use.
3 Squirt the desired amount onto a cotton pad – 3 squirts should do the trick – and cleanse in circular motions.
4 No need to wash off post use.

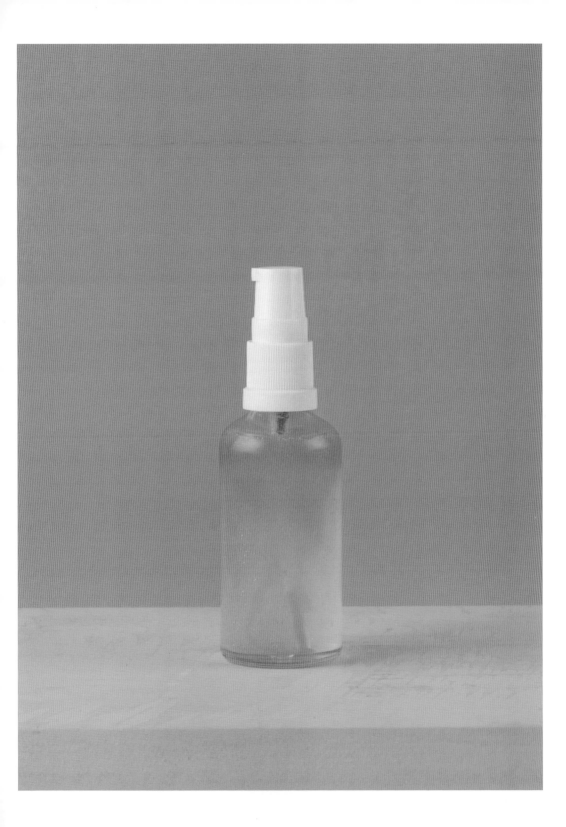

A *Rosehip* by any other name does not smell as sweet

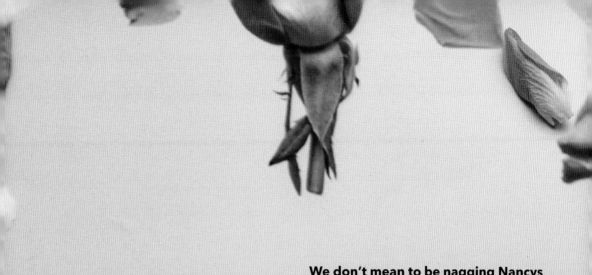

We don't mean to be nagging Nancys over here but we'll say it again: read your labels!

They will reveal quickly whether you're getting bang for your buck. The INCI, which denotes the scientific name for a cosmetic ingredient, for the almighty scar-healing and rejuvenating rosehip oil is Rosa Mosqueta or Rosa Rubiginosa, from the rose plant grown in Chile. It's friendly neighbour Rosa Canina is often slipped in as a cheaper and more widely available substitute in beauty products and even by companies selling 'pure' rosehip oil. While it's a great hydrating oil that acts an emollient on the skin, it does not contain any of the healing properties of Rosa Rubiginosa, and is far less expensive to produce. When you're paying top dollar for your rosehip, make sure you're getting the right one.

aftersun soothing balm

6g shea butter
3g beeswax
15ml oat oil
3ml macerated carrot
  tissue oil
2 drops chamomile
  essential oil

————————

MAKES:
30g

SHELF LIFE:
6 months in an airtight
container.

HELPFUL HINT:
You can blend in some aloe
at point of use for extra anti-
inflammatory benefits.

If you've caught a bit of sun, this one is a real winner. Oat oil is rich in oleic acid, which has a moisturising and regenerating effect on the skin. Carrot oil is high in beta-carotenes, and there is increasing evidence that carotenoids protect the skin against photo-oxidative sun damage. Shea butter and beeswax are incredibly moisturising and enhance the skin's elasticity and flexibility, acting as a shield against external aggressors such as cold, sun, salt water or wind. Slather this all over if you're pink in the cheeks. Chamomile is an anti-inflammatory essential oil and makes a wonderful treatment for soothing painful burns. Don't forget your SPF next time!

————————

1 Melt the shea butter and beeswax in a bain-marie until liquid.
2 Add the oat and carrot oils.
3 Cool then add the chamomile essential oil.
4 Pour into your container to cool completely.
5 Use as often as needed after sun exposure.

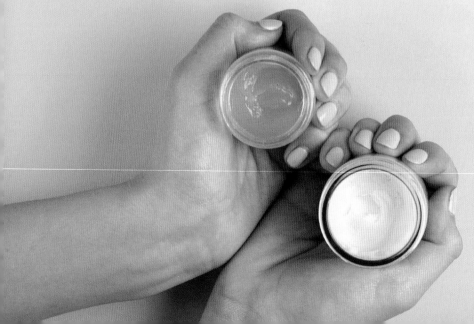

the home run

5g beeswax
20g shea butter
20ml argan oil
4ml honey
1 drop vitamin E oil

————————

MAKES:
50g

SHELF LIFE:
6 months in an airtight
container. Only apply with
a scoop or clean hands.

HELPFUL HINT:
Vitamin E is added not
only for its moisturising
properties, but also to
slow down the rancidity
of the oils.

This is a rich winter balm for use on dry, chapped skin. The
ingredients of butters, oils and honey are ultra nourishing,
hydrating and offer protection against wind and cold. The balm
can be used on the face and lips, but also works a dream on
your dry body bits like elbows and cuticles. It is what we like
to call an all-rounder and our personal stash tends to hang
around in our handbags. Argan oil isn't just great for your hair;
it has a high natural fatty acid and vitamin E content, but it is
also non-pore-clogging and non-greasy (non-comedogenic, as
the science buffs like to say), so makes a great addition to facial
concoctions. Honey will attract moisture and keep it in the skin,
and is soothing and moisturising for tender dry skin. Lather up!

————————

1 Melt down the wax and butter until liquid in a bain-marie.
2 Use a cold bath to slowly cool the mixture while adding the oil,
honey and vitamin E.
3 Once it traces with a spoon, decant into a container.
4 Leave to cool at room temperature.

crease-away eye serum

20ml grapeseed oil
9ml olive squalane
5ml pomegranate seed oil
1 drop vitamin E oil

MAKES:
35ml

SHELF LIFE:
6 months in an airtight container.

HELPFUL HINT:
When buying your squalane, most commonly derived from olive oil, make sure it's not squalene (spot the e!), as this is shark liver oil.

The area around the eyes needs to be treated with extra gentleness; the potency of some active ingredients and essential oils can irritate the fine skin, but it is the part of the face most prone to dryness and continued dryness can lead to signs of ageing (i.e. the dreaded crow's feet). Keep the area hydrated and supple with this luxurious blend of oils, perfect to keep any pesky lines, feet or other, at bay. Grapeseed is rich in tannins, as well as vitamin E, so it's the perfect foundation to tone and firm the skin. Squalane, a hydrating agent derived from olives, is lightweight and penetrates deeply to improve the skin's elasticity. It also has humectant properties, which help maintain optimum moisture levels in the skin. Pomegranate is a potent anti-inflammatory, which is fab for puffy eyes and under-eye bags, while helping to reduce the appearance of wrinkles and fine lines. It also smells deeeeeeee-lish.

---

1 Blend the oils and squalane.
2 Add the vitamin E.
3 Mix vigorously before decanting into your container.

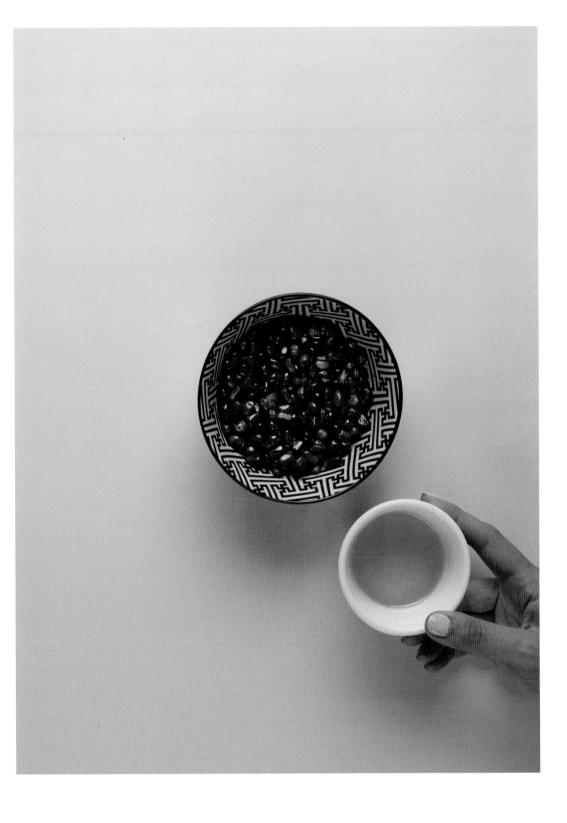

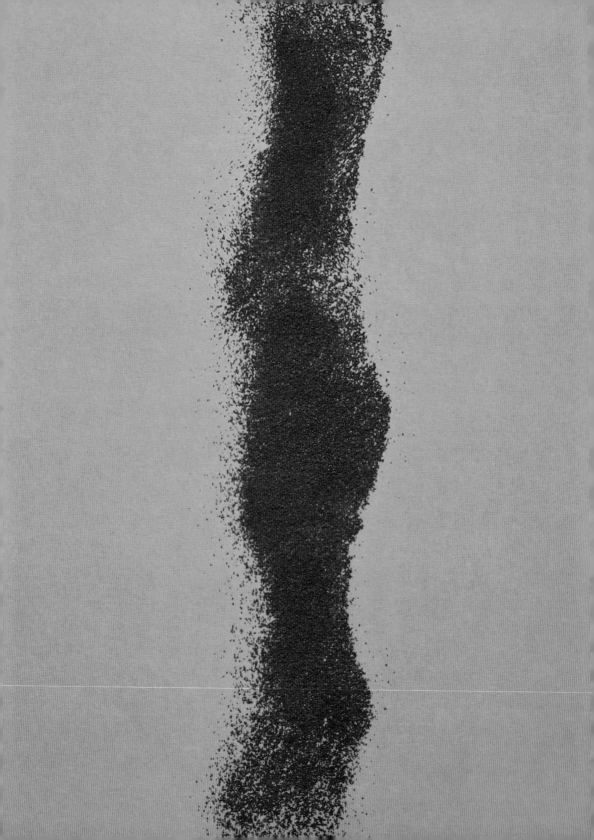

jojoba? ooh la la

10ml jojoba oil
5 drops lavender
   essential oil
20g jojoba beads
5g dried lavender

MAKES:
30ml

SHELF LIFE:
3 months; 6 without the
dried flowers.

HELPFUL HINT:
If using in the shower, keep
wet fingers out as it can
speed up the expiry of the
product.

Conventional facial scrubs use microbeads for the abrasive, exfoliating action on the skin. Aside from the fact that these are bad for the environment, rubbing plastic all over your face isn't really a great idea. The good news is that there are tons of natural abrasive exfoliators and jojoba beads are a firm favourite at CBCo HQ. They are bright blue, made from jojoba wax, and they remove dead skin cells and impurities, leaving a glowing complexion. Mixed with lavender and jojoba oils, the blend is soothing and calming for the skin post scrub.

---

1 Combine the oil and essential oil.
2 Stir in the jojoba beads and dried lavender.
3 Decant into a container.

cheeky stain

9g cocoa butter
7g beeswax
13ml grapeseed oil
1g coloured pigment

MAKES:
30g

SHELF LIFE:
6 months. Apply with clean hands.

HELPFUL HINT:
Grapeseed oil is a cost-effective oil used in many natural cosmetics, but swap it with any other light carrier oils if you don't have any to hand.

This beauty is a naturally coloured stain for your lips or cheeks. Ingredients with a coloured pigment are the way to go when creating stains. Your mica powders, natural oxides and natural powders like beetroot or pink hibiscus flower will create your ideal colour and depth, depending on how dramatic or subtle you want the stain. We've put together a basic formula from which you can experiment with colour, as long as the ratio of ingredients remains the same.

---

1 Melt the butter and wax in a bain-marie.
2 Blend in the oil.
3 Stir in the coloured pigment to reach the desired colour and depth.
4 Decant into your container.

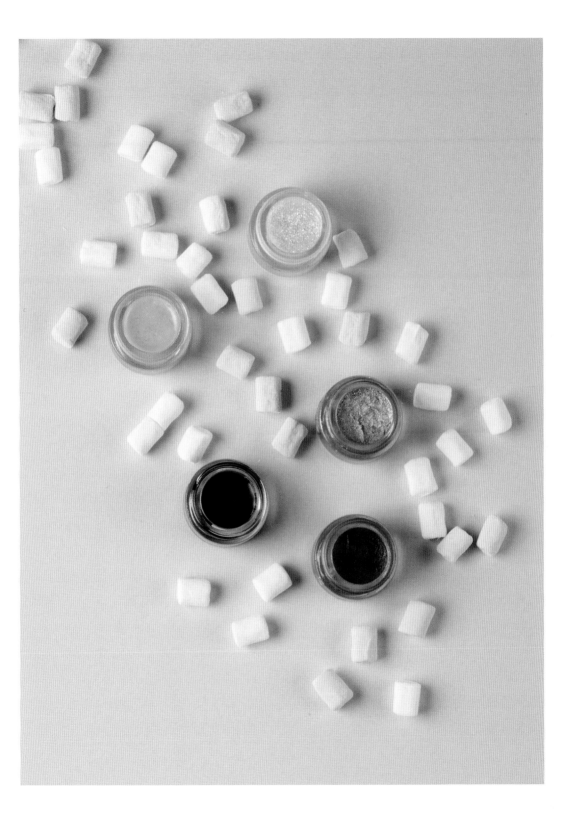

skin-clearing toner

1 drop willow bark extract (vegetable salicylic acid)
49ml witch hazel hydrosol
3 drops tea tree essential oil

MAKES:
50ml

SHELF LIFE:
3 months; if using pre-preserved witch hazel hydrosol. If not, up to 1 week if kept in the fridge.

HELPFUL HINT:
Tea tree essential oil can be applied directly to the skin, however give the toner a good shake before use to ensure even distribution.

Spots got you down? Chin up, babe, we've got a toner that will clear any blemishes right up. Willow bark extract, or vegetable salicylic acid, is a beta hydroxy acid (BHA) and a keratolytic agent, which promotes the shedding of dead skin layers and skin renewal. It's astringent and antibacterial, so helps to fight imperfections and regulate the sebum in the skin. Witch hazel is perfect for congested skin as it's anti-inflammatory, antiseptic and cooling for the skin. Use up to 5 per cent salicylic acid and you could keep it in the fridge for an extra cooling and refreshing sensation.

---

1 Stir the willow bark extract into the hydrosol.
2 Add your essential oil.
3 Decant into a spray bottle.
4 Use as a toner on congested skin.

see ya spot gel

1 drop rosemary essential oil
1 drop thyme essential oil
1 drop cypress essential oil
5ml jojoba oil
15g aloe vera gel

Aloe vera, considered by the Egyptians to be the plant of immortality, is known to have many healing properties, including relief from dry and damaged skin. It can treat infection and is an anti-inflammatory, making it a powerful tool when dealing with pesky spots. We've mixed with jojoba oil to form a thick gel. Add your essential oils, which contain antimicrobial, antiseptic and antibacterial properties, and it will zap any problems in no time.

MAKES:
20g

SHELF LIFE:
4–6 weeks in the fridge if using preserved aloe; if not, up to 1 week.

HELPFUL HINT:
These essential oils pack a powerful punch and should only be used in combination to treat spots and acne, avoiding the eye area.

1 Blend the essential oils and jojoba oil.
2 Stir in the aloe vera gel.
3 Decant into a container.
4 Dab onto spots directly using clean fingers.

mmm cappuccino lips

5ml honey
4ml castor oil
10g ground coffee
1 drop vanilla extract

_____

MAKES:
20g

SHELF LIFE:
3 months in an airtight
container.

HELPFUL HINT:
Pop it on a toothbrush to
get extra exfoliating lip
action!

Who says your lips don't need a good scrubbing occasionally?
Ever tried to apply lipstick to dry and flaky lips? Yeah, we hear
ya! The caffeine provides a temporary plumping effect, just as it
does on skin, so it's a neat inclusion in your lip scrub. The honey
and castor oil will ensure that post scrubbing, your lips remain
moisturised, soft and shiny. Vanilla is there to improve the taste,
as it is pretty close to your mouth – chances are the odd flake
will fall in!

_____

1 Mix the honey and oil together.
2 Add the coffee to form a thick paste.
3 Add the vanilla extract for taste and smell.

fresh 'n' floral

10ml jojoba oil
10ml macadamia nut oil
10ml sweet almond oil
2 drops lavender essential
  oil
2 drops geranium
  essential oil
1 drop vitamin E oil

Serums are all the rage these days, and here at CBCo, we're mega fans of oil-based face serums. The key is to keep the blends light, with oils that absorb quickly into the skin so that the skin can drink up the potent active botanicals in the natural nut, seed and plant oils. This serum has a wonderful floral scent from the gentle essential oils, which are both skin enhancers and toners. The oils are light, and aim to balance the skin's natural sebum. A common misconception is that oils make the skin oily, but, in fact, quite the opposite is true: oils help to calm overactive glands and level out imbalances, making oily skin *less* oily. Who woulda thunk it?!

MAKES:
30ml

SHELF LIFE:
6 months in an airtight
container.

HELPFUL HINT:
Keep serums in sterilised,
dark bottles to slow
down the oxidation and
preserve the potency of the
ingredients.

1 Blend all the carrier oils together.
2 Add the essential oils.
3 Decant into a dark pump bottle.

get your rosy glow

**45ml floral water of
  your choice
5ml barbary fig oil**

MAKES:
50ml

SHELF LIFE:
3 months with a pre-
preserved floral water; up to
1 week in the fridge if not.

HELPFUL HINT:
Store in the fridge for an
extra cooling sensation.

There's nothing more refreshing than a spritz of our fav
rosewater toner fresh from the fridge. Get Your Rosy Glow goes
down an absolute storm at our workshops and the great thing
about a two-ingredient recipe is that it's super-easy to customise.
We encourage you to keep the barbary fig oil for two reasons:
1) it's suited to most skin types and, 2) when mixed with a
floral water and shaken, it looks like a bottle of glitter. We love
the sparkles. If rose doesn't tickle your fancy, there's a ton of
floral waters you can experiment with for scent and feeling,
depending on your skin type.

1 Decant your floral water into a container.
2 Add in your oil.
3 Shake well before use.

Floral Water: We love getting creative with the scents of the floral
waters that we use. Try combining the sweet scents of Orange
Blossom and Rose for an uplifting spritz, or the decadent tones of
Jasmine and Geranium Rose for a relaxing spray. If you're looking
for a soothing and subtle option then Chamomile and Lavender is
a lovely combo, while Witch Hazel and Rosemary will stimulate tired
minds. We also use our Rosy Glow as a multi-purpose product; sure,
its a wonderful skin brightener but it is also fab as a yoga spray, body
spritz, room scent and we've even been to known to put a quick
pump on our pillow to help us sleep at night. Refer to Hydrosols on
p. 24 for further inspiration.

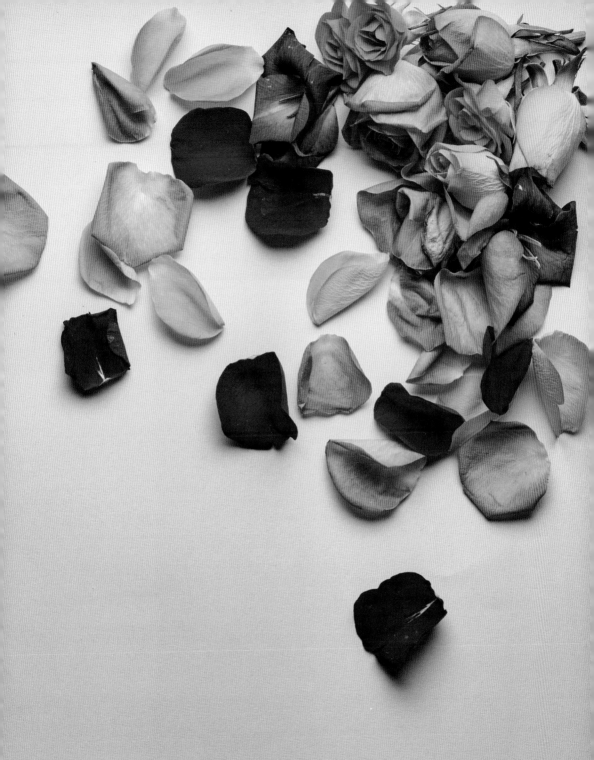

forever-young serum

15ml jojoba oil
10ml rosehip oil
5ml olive squalane
5ml pomegranate seed oil
2 drops frankincense
   essential oil

_____

MAKES:
30ml

SHELF LIFE:
6 months in an airtight
container.

HELPFUL HINT:
You can add other floral
essential oils for fragrance
here, like geranium or
lavender. Use a maximum
of 4 drops per 30ml.

This serum is a wonderful blend of the best regenerating and
rejuvenating oils to promote supple, youthful skin and to protect
against the free radicals that can contribute to premature
ageing. Squalane is a powerful emollient; it softens the skin
and improves elasticity, reducing the appearance of ageing.
Pomegranate seed oil contains high levels of antioxidants,
which help to prevent damage caused by environmental toxins.
Frankincense essential oil helps to reduce the appearance of sun
damage, age spots or skin discolorations.

_____

1 Blend the carrier oils together.
2 Add the essential oil.
3 Decant into a dark pump bottle.

bathe like an egyptian

25g oatmeal
25g rice bran powder
25g ground almond meal
25g coconut milk powder

MAKES:
100g

SHELF LIFE:
6 months, as long as no
water enters the dry mixture.

HELPFUL HINT:
Use food-grade, organic
ingredients where possible.

Bathing in oats and milk, Cleopatra knew she was on to a good thing. This gentle exfoliating milk can be used in place of your regular foamy cleanser. It's incredibly anti-inflammatory, moisturising and soothing, and all the ingredients are great gentle exfoliators, rich in essential fatty acids and vitamin E. When mixed with water, the mixture will create a silky milky water that will wipe away dirt, grime and make-up. You could also mix with milk, to get the benefits of naturally occurring lactic acid, which is great for sloughing away dead skin cells. This cleanser is particularly good for sensitive skin where typical cleansers are too drying.

---

1 Combine all the ingredients together and transfer to a container.
2 To use, mix enough powder for your face with equal parts of water in a small bowl to create the milk.
3 Apply with your (clean!) fingers and use a damp muslin cloth to remove any residue.

panda eyes

20ml EcoSilk
15ml camellia seed oil
10ml castor oil
4ml olive oil
1 drop vitamin E oil

MAKES:
50ml

SHELF LIFE:
6 months in an airtight container.

HELPFUL HINT:
Keep serums in sterilised, dark bottles to slow down the oxidation and preserve the potency of the ingredients.

Most eye make-up is oil-based, so trying to remove it with anything water-based will prove quite difficult! This blend of oils and emollients is particularly good for use around the gentle eye area, and all are safe in case you get any in your eye. If you can get your hands on some EcoSilk, it can be added to a blend of oils to make a fantastic moisturising eye make-up remover. Emollients soften the skin and EcoSilk is made from renewable natural sources such as sugar and coconut; it moisturises but also makes the remover more spreadable. Camellia seed oil is a natural plant oil, normally grown in Japan, that contains antioxidants and polyphenols that help to revitalise the skin. Castor oil is thought to promote hair growth and thickening, so slather this baby on your lashes and eyebrows! It also promotes collagen and elastin production in the skin. This is an eye make-up remover and eye serum in one; we're seriously winning on the efficiency front with this one! Thank us later, guys, thank us later.

---

1 Blend all the oils, including the EcoSilk, together.
2 Add the vitamin E.
3 Stir well and decant into a dark pump bottle.

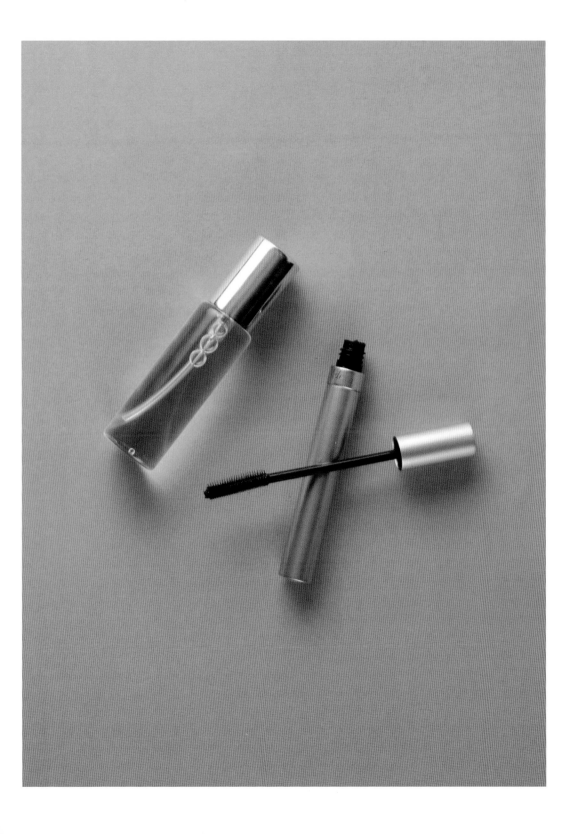

Made *up*

We get asked about natural make-up a lot.

We have to admit we dabble in a bit of DIY cosmetics but decided to leave most of it to the experts. Finding a way to create pigment, colour, shimmer and shine without adding harsh chemicals is easier said than done, but luckily for us there are some fantastic brands out there dedicated to doing just that. Granted, natural make-up does a slightly different job than high-street alternatives because frankly it's not natural to have lipstick that stays on your lips for 12 hours straight. Just imagine what goes into it to achieve that... So you will find that you have to reapply a little more but other than that, everything from a smoky eye to a dewy glow is achievable with the brands that are on the market these days. We've rounded up the best of the bunch (and trust us, we've tried our fair share) – super-cool brands using advanced formulation and nourishing, non-toxic ingredients.

RMS Beauty: An amazing range of cosmetics that's available to buy across the country. Founded by make-up artist Rose-Marie Swift who, after discovering her blood contained high levels of heavy metals from years of continual exposure to beauty products that were rich in things like lead and aluminium, decided to switch to all-natural alternatives and ultimately created her own line. RMS is filled with creamy foundations, amazing concealers, lipsticks, cheek balms and their all new 'master mixer', which has been featured in the beauty press across the globe as it basically makes you look like a shining, golden goddess. *www.rmsbeauty.com*

Jane Iredale: A line dedicated to making mineral make-up. Incredibly multi-functional, it provides great results while also being good for the skin. They do some killer foundations and we especially love their primer, which helps set foundation while providing a dewy finish. Our all-time fave is the brow kit: we're lovers of a brow here at CBCo and this kit has everything you need to make Miss Delevingne herself envious. *www.janeiredale.com*

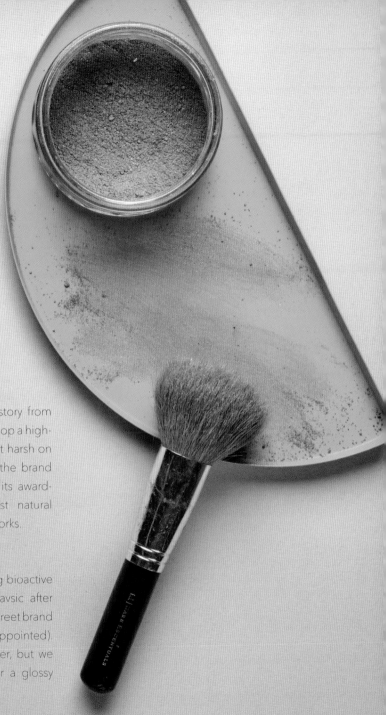

Kjaer Weis: Yet another inspiring story from founder Kirsten, who looked to develop a high-performing cosmetic line that wasn't harsh on women's skin. Eight years on and the brand has achieved cult status thanks to its award-winning foundations and the first natural mascara we've found that actually works. *www.kjaerweis.com*

ILIA: A super-sleek range containing bioactive ingredients, founded by Sasha Plavsic after doing some research into her high-street brand of lipstick (and being pretty disappointed). These guys do lipsticks like no other, but we especially love their Multi-sticks for a glossy finish for lips, eyes and cheeks. *www.iliabeauty.com*

Fries before guys.

body

total babe body butter

50g mango butter
50ml jojoba oil
5 drops geranium
   essential oil
2 drops vitamin E oil

MAKES:
100g

SHELF LIFE:
6 months in an airtight
container.

HELPFUL HINT:
Adding shimmer or glitter
(biodegradable, if possible)
to this turns a simple body
butter into a fab gift as well.

This is a great body butter recipe that's light enough to use every day, but will still give a good kick of moisture and nourishment: basically an all-round babe for your skin. We've gone for a 50/50 split of butter to oil, which gives it a lotion-like consistency, without needing to add any water. Mango butter is a great healing butter; it contains vitamin A, linolenic and fatty acids, which all contribute to accelerating the healing of skin conditions while also being incredibly moisturising. Jojoba oil is a general winner and doesn't get its praises sung as much as it should. It's the oil that's closest to the structure of human sebum oil — the oil that your skin naturally produces to keep skin cleansed and healthy. The production of this is also linked to acne, so jojoba is fantastic at balancing and evening out any spotty or breakout areas. We've popped in some geranium, as it's a great antibacterial option that helps to improve blood circulation just below the skin, in turn improving the appearance of any patchy, dry or uneven areas.

1 Melt the mango butter in a bain-marie.
2 Slowly add the jojoba oil, stirring as you do.
3 Place in the fridge to cool for 5 minutes.
4 Stir in the essential oils.
5 Whisk the mixture with an electric whisk, then put back in the fridge for a further 5 minutes.
6 Repeat until you have a creamy texture, almost like icing on a cake.
7 Spoon into your container, being careful to maintain the fluffiness.

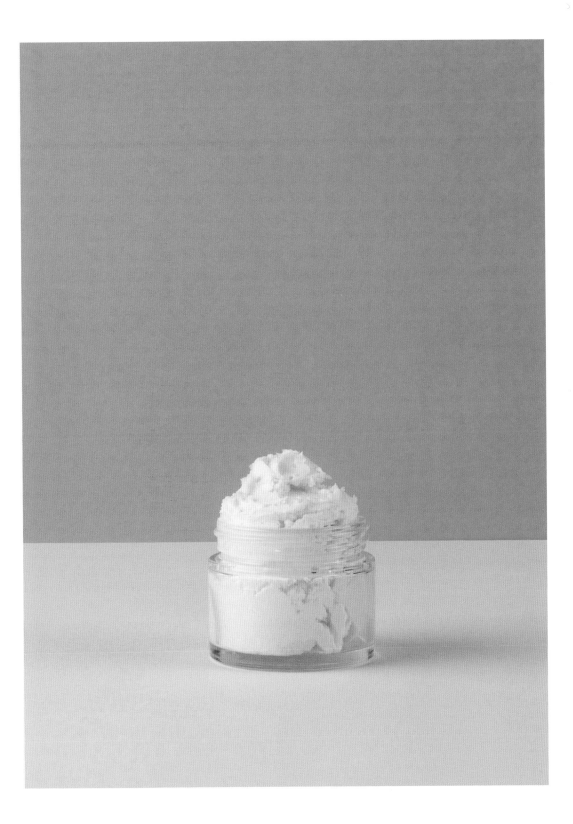

detox and purify bath soak

10 drops lavender
   essential oil
10 drops peppermint
   essential oil
20ml evening primrose oil
100g Epsom salts
80g pink Himalayan salt

MAKES:
200g

SHELF LIFE:
6 months stored in an
airtight container.

HELPFUL HINT:
This may make your bath
slippery! Be sure to take care
when getting in or out of the
bath. The quantity should
make enough for 4 baths;
you can make in bigger
batches if needed.

Sometimes your skin needs a good old detox in the same way that your body does after a heavy weekend. This amazingly powerful bath soak is perfect for giving your skin and mind an overhaul; we recommend using it on a Sunday evening so that you're in a great state of mind for the following week. Both the Epsom and pink salts have absorbent properties and will draw impurities and toxins out of the skin. Evening primrose is an antioxidant, helping to calm skin and improve the appearance of lines and age spots. Finally, lavender and peppermint give this an exhilarating fragrance that will bring an element of focus and calm to the mind.

---

1 Add your essential oils to the evening primrose oil and stir well.
2 Combine with both salts.
3 Store in an airtight jar and add a scoop to a running bath to use.

zest espresso

150g ground coffee
30g pink Himalayan salt
20ml sweet almond oil
5 drops tangerine
  essential oil

MAKES:
200g

SHELF LIFE:
3 months in an airtight
container. Keep wet fingers
out so the shelf life doesn't
become compromised.
Instead, use a spoon or
scoop to take out some of
the scrub.

HELPFUL HINT:
The longer you can keep
this scrub on the skin before
washing off the better;
5–10 minutes will allow the
caffeine to activate and
penetrate the skin further.
Plump skin awaits you!

Just wait until you smell this baby! The combination of coffee
and tangerine has such a powerful scent that we challenge you
not to want to eat it (please don't, though, we're not convinced
it'll taste as good as it smells). The addition of the Himalayan salt
is perfect for detoxifying; this salt is high in minerals and nutrients
that are released as it's mixed with warm water, meaning your
skin will really feel the benefits. The salt is also great for soothing
tired muscles and easing joint and muscle tension. The tangerine
is a milder member of the citrus essential oil crew and therefore
makes it suitable even for super-sensitive souls. The chemical
composition of the oil is known to help reduce fluid retention, in
turn minimising the appearance of bumps and unsightly stretch
marks. That, combined with the vitamin E in the sweet almond
oil, helps to smooth and brighten while leaving skin moisturised
and hydrated. Enjoy!

---

1 Combine the coffee and salt.
2 In a separate bowl, mix the almond and tangerine oils.
3 Combine both mixtures and stir well to ensure the oil is evenly
distributed.
4 Can be used either on dry skin pre-showering or on wet skin
during your shower.

OHEMGEE we love fuss free

70g coconut oil
30ml carrier oil of
   your choice
2 drops vitamin E oil

MAKES:
100g

SHELF LIFE:
6 months, but keep wet
fingers out if you're keeping
it in the shower.

HELPFUL HINT:
Don't let your mixture reach
too high a temperature as
this could make it grainy
when it solidifies.

Our fuss-free body moisturiser has reached legendary status in CBCo households. We have aunties requesting weekly batches to help with eczema, boyfriends nagging us for new tubs to soothe shaving rash and friends begging for more to keep their pins super smooth. It all began with a simple experiment: can we create an in-shower moisturiser using all natural ingredients? We called upon our dear friend coconut oil and started experimenting. The result: a rich, luxurious, multi-purpose balm that's super-easy to use. We're all aware of the benefits of coconut oil by now: it's super-high in fatty acids with a molecular structure that allows it to penetrate skin and hair in a way that other oils can't. Even once it's been rinsed off the skin, the moisture stays locked in, which makes for a superb in-shower moisturiser. Slather it on, rinse it off, no need to moisturise once you're out and dry. We've popped in both jojoba and rosehip oils for an anti-inflammatory and highly antioxidant combination. We're going to talk you through how to customise this one as it's super-simple, all you need is to follow the ingredient split that we've outlined for you.

---

1 Melt the coconut oil in a bain-marie.
2 Once liquid, add you carrier oils, vitamin E oil and essential oils (if using) and stir well.
3 Decant into an airtight jar and store in the fridge until the mixture solidifies into a balm.
4 Use on the body or face as a balm or wash-off moisturiser.

Carrier Oil: Get creative here. Jojoba, rosehip, sweet almond, olive, argan, peach kernel… or a combination of two or three. If you find coconut oil quite heavy then mix it with something lighter, such as macadamia nut oil, to make it more suitable for your skin. Refer to Carrier Oils 101 (p. 22) for inspiration.

Optional: Ten drops of your essential oil of choice. Again, go crazy. This is going to be what fragrances your balm. A mix of citrus essential oils works well (grapefruit, tangerine, lemon) and is really refreshing to use in the morning. You might fancy a luxurious combination of frankincense and helichrysum that'll be great for more mature skin. Or stay simple with lavender, which is wonderful for dry skin and areas of eczema. Refer to Essential Oils 101 (p. 26) for more ideas.

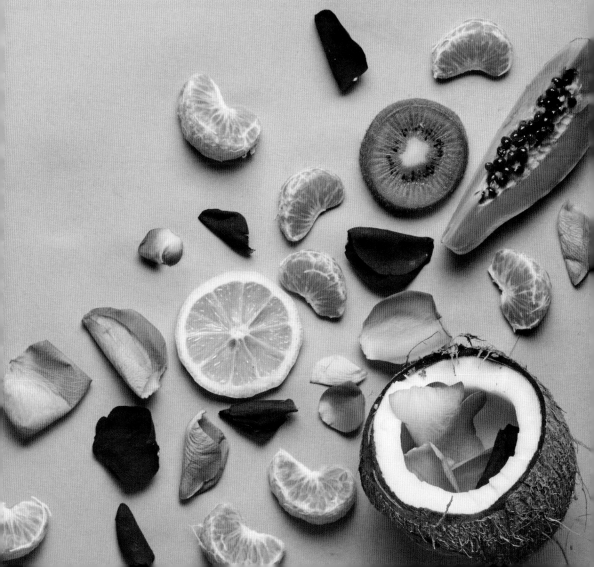

frappuccino bars

85g shea butter
80g ground coffee
85g coconut oil
5 drops geranium
 essential oil
5 drops grapefruit
 essential oil

MAKES:
10 bars

SHELF LIFE:
6 months in an airtight
container.

HELPFUL HINT:
Why not mix things up a bit
and use a shaped muffin
tray? We love heart shapes.

Our coffee scrubs are by far our most popular recipes (see p. 72 and p. 157 for other scrubs). People have cottoned on to how fantastic coffee is as an exfoliator and how damn easy it is to throw one together. So we wanted to give you a next-level recipe for something snazzy once you've mastered the basics. We've decided to rejig our fabulous scrub to a little bar that is just the right size for one full body scrub – waste not, want not – and perfect for a quick post-gym shower. They're compact but still pack a serious punch. We don't need to tell you about the benefits coffee has on the appearance of your skin (we're looking at you, cellulite) as we've talked about that earlier in the book, but the added benefit of these bars is the butter. Incredibly moisturising and high in vitamin E, it'll leave your scrubbed skin super-soft. Grapefruit and geranium are a pretty powerful combo: both help to stimulate blood flow and circulation, which, when combined with the coffee, will give you one hell of a kick in the morning.

---

1 Divide the shea butter in two and put one half to one side.
2 Melt the other half in a bain-marie.
3 Add the coffee and stir well, then spoon the mixture into a small, silicone muffin tray; we use a 3 × 3cm tray.
4 Leave a gap at the top of each, the idea being the coconut oil will sit on top and form a white layer, and place in the freezer to cool.
5 Melt down the coconut oil and the remaining shea butter in a bain-marie.
6 Add the essential oils and stir well.
7 Once the coffee is solid, remove from the freezer.
8 Pour the liquid coconut mixture on top of each 'muffin'.
9 Place in the fridge and again allow the entire mixture to solidify.
10 Keep in the fridge and use as and when you need.

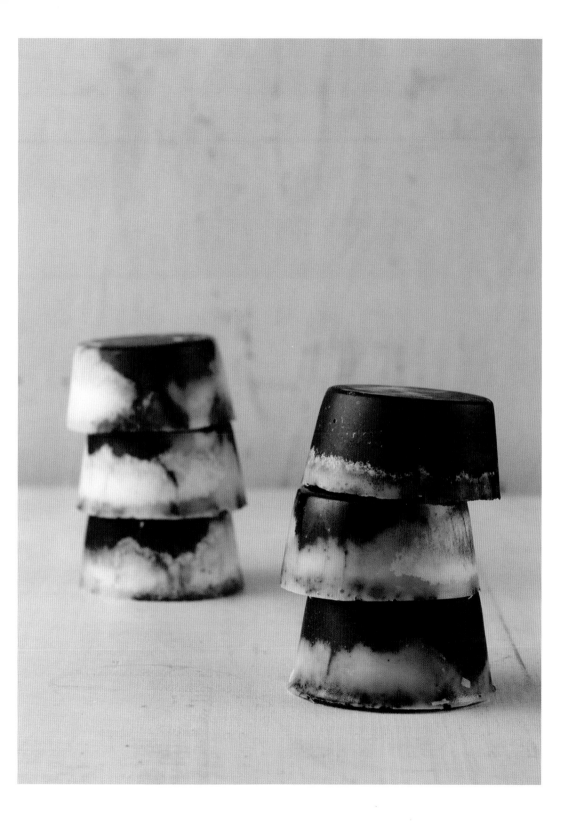

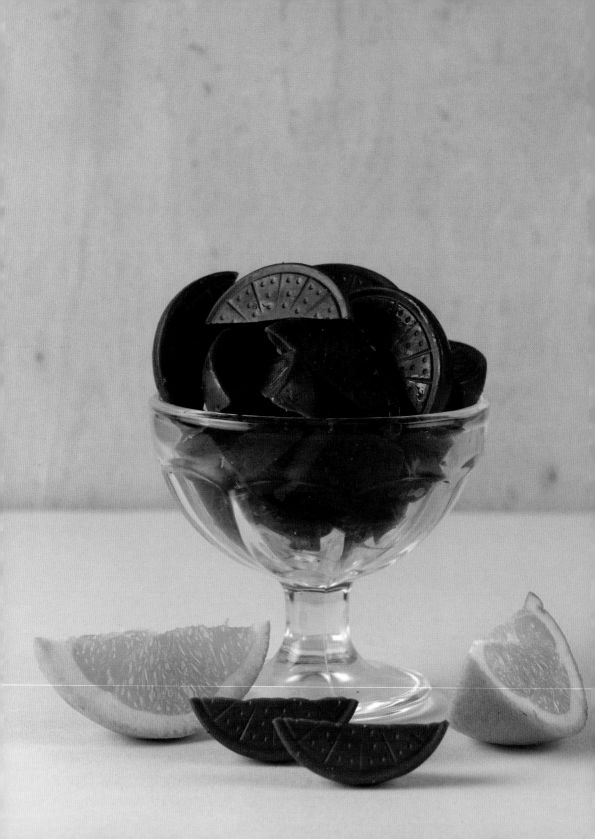

chocolate orange
bath melts

50g cocoa butter
25g coconut oil
5 drops tangerine
   essential oil
5 drops sweet orange
   essential oil

MAKES:
75g

SHELF LIFE:
6 months in an airtight
container.

HELPFUL HINT:
Keep in the fridge or in a
cool place or they can melt.

These are absolutely wonderful for one of those end-of-day, long and luxurious baths that literally melt away your worries. A bit of 'me' time, which we all need now and again. The great thing about these little melts is that they'll make your bath smell delightful, while leaving your body super-moisturised and you won't need to apply moisturiser when you get out the bath: all that lovely hydration stays locked in even after rinsing. Tangerine and sweet orange essential oils will give this the citric kick, a bit like a chocolate orange, but they are also extremely antioxidising, which helps to keep skin firm and youthful.

1 Melt the cocoa butter in a bain-marie.
2 Add the coconut oil until both are liquid form.
3 Add the essential oils and stir well.
4 Decant into a small, silicone muffin tray and place in the fridge until they have fully solidified.
5 Store in the fridge and simply take out when you fancy a bathtime treat.
6 Add to a bath under hot running water and allow to melt.

let's be firm

70ml rosehip oil
30ml apricot kernel oil
5 drops cypress
  essential oil
5 drops frankincense
  essential oil

MAKES:
100ml

SHELF LIFE:
6 months stored in an
airtight container.

HELPFUL HINT:
This can also be used on
the face as a powerful night
serum.

Whether you're curvaceous and full-figured, a six-foot size six or anything in between, there is sure to be an area of your body that you wish was that teeny tiny bit firmer. We're throwing aside the fact that you are probably the ONLY one who notices any wobbly bits, because you're obviously absolutely gorgeous as you are, but we know you'll insist that your thighs are definitely a little cuddly so we're sharing our favourite body-firming serum. The secret here is including ingredients that are high in omega fatty acids to replace suppleness, have astringent properties to tighten the top layer of skin and are antioxidising to promote both cell renewal and blood flow, in turn giving the skin a younger and firmer appearance. Rosehip is often used in firming recipes, due to its high content of essential fatty acids, omegas and vitamin E. We love the texture as it's incredibly rich but not greasy. We're also adding apricot kernel oil, which brings high levels of vitamin C – another powerful antioxidant. Cypress and frankincense are both strong astringents, meaning they have a tightening effect on the top layer of the skin, as well as being detoxifying and promoting healthy circulation.

---

1 Combine the rosehip and apricot oils.
2 Add both essential oils and stir well to ensure they are evenly distributed.
3 Decant and store in a dark glass bottle.
4 Use after showering for best results.

cool down aftersun

40ml peppermint hydrosol
35ml chamomile hydrosol
10ml aloe vera gel
5ml vegetable glycerine

MAKES:
100ml

SHELF LIFE:
3 months if using pre-preserved floral waters; if not, store in the fridge and use within 1 week.

HELPFUL HINT:
It's also possible to use aloe vera powder, simply dissolve in the hydrosols.

We obviously need to stress that we do not encourage going out in the sun without sunscreen. It is not a good idea. Both UVA and UVB rays are incredibly damaging to the skin and will ultimately disrupt cell renewal, as well as possibly doing much worse. However, we do know that there are times when you simply get caught out and there's no avoiding that. So we've thrown together a cooling spray that will help to soothe tender areas of sunburn and speed up the healing process. Aloe is an age-old sunburn healer due to its powerful antioxidant qualities and its ability to calm inflamed and angry skin. We've combined it with peppermint hydrosol for an instant cooling fix as well as chamomile hydrosol to reduce redness. Finally, the addition of glycerine injects some much-needed moisture.

1 Combine the waters with the aloe vera gel and stir well until the latter is evenly distributed.
2 Add the glycerine and stir again.
3 Store in a mist spray bottle and shake well before each use.

Sunscreen-off:

While we're obviously all about the DIY, we do not recommend making your own sunscreen.

It's very difficult to achieve proper SPF broad-spectrum protection, and particularly equal zinc distribution, without expensive scientific equipment. If the zinc isn't adequately distributed you risk parts of the skin being unprotected and there's no way of testing the SPF protection at home unless you go outside and see if you burn. Not a good idea! When we're buying our sunscreens, we favour mineral-based sunscreens rather than traditional chemical sunscreens. Yes, we hear your resounding WHY? Tell us more!

Chemical sunscreens work by using a combination of chemicals that, when mixed and activated, create a reaction that stops the skin from burning under UV rays. Mineral sunscreens are made up of just that – minerals – which act as a physical block sitting on top of the skin, reflecting the rays. We look specifically for mineral combinations of titanium dioxide and uncoated non-nano zinc oxide to provide broad-spectrum protection against UVA and UVB rays. Chemical sunscreens typically take time to activate once applied, but can also contain harsher chemicals that strip your skin of their natural sheen. They aren't great for the environment either: they aren't biodegradable, so they slip off you and into the ocean where they remain to be gobbled up by fish and other marine life.

Natural sunscreens have come a long way since the days of the thick and gloopy white substance that didn't tend to absorb well. Rather than red-faced, they left you rather ghostly. Luckily, there are now some wonderful brands making lightweight and nourishing mineral sunscreens. If you're after a gentler, natural alternative, brands such as John Masters, Jason and Green People are all non-toxic, fragrance-free and we promise they won't hide your tan!

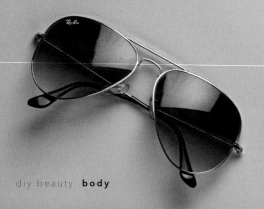

chemical
vs mineral

While we're on the topic, sunscreen is the hands-down best thing you can do for your skin. Wear sunscreen, like all the time. Well, maybe not to bed, but seriously every other time. UV rays destroy the cells in your skin that lead to regeneration, so the effect won't show now, but it will in later life when your skin loses its ability to replicate and the collagen and elastin are depleted. Happens with age, unfortunately, we know it's a bummer. UV rays can penetrate your skin if it's sunny, if it's raining, if it's overcast or if it's grey. Wearing at least SPF 20 everyday will do so much more for your skin than any cream or serum will.

You won't see the benefits now, but trust us, you'll thank us later. Sunscreen is also one of the products we advise leaving to the experts rather than attempting yourself.

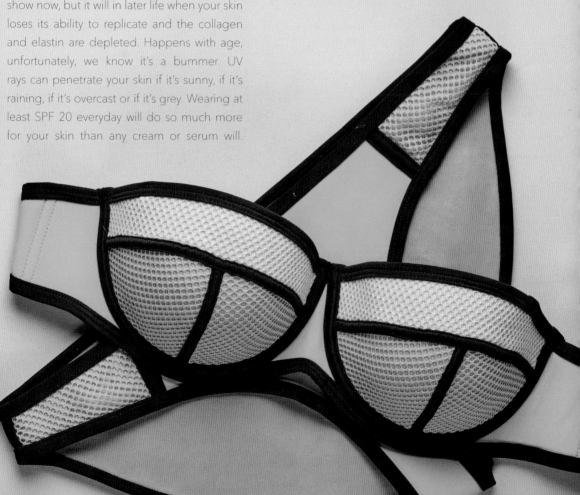

pull-up paws

5g shea butter
10g coconut oil
10ml jojoba oil
25g cane sugar
5 drops lemon essential
    oil

MAKES:
50g

SHELF LIFE:
6 months in an airtight
container.

HELPFUL HINT:
Follow up with our Total
Babe Body Butter (p. 154)
for an extra-moisturising hit.

If you're anything like us, you love a good play on the gym monkey bars. We're often sulking about trying to do pull-ups (failing), Olympic lifts (better) and handstands (killer). All of these slick moves take a toll on your paws and we're often left with dry, calloused claws that are totally not sexy. So along with scrubbing the rest of our bods, we like to put something special together for our hands. A good hand scrub goes a long way, particularly during winter, when our hands also tend to get super-dry. We're using sugar, coconut oil and lemon to slough away rough skin, swipe away pesky bacteria and make sure your hands are clean and supple. The added shea butter will continue to moisturise and protect into your next gym session to make sure your hands stay less claw, more satin.

---

1   Melt the shea butter in a bain-marie.
2   Mix in the coconut and jojoba oils.
3   Allow to cool, and then stir in the sugar and essential oil.
4   Decant into a container.
5   Use a coin-shaped amount for a good all-over hand scrub.

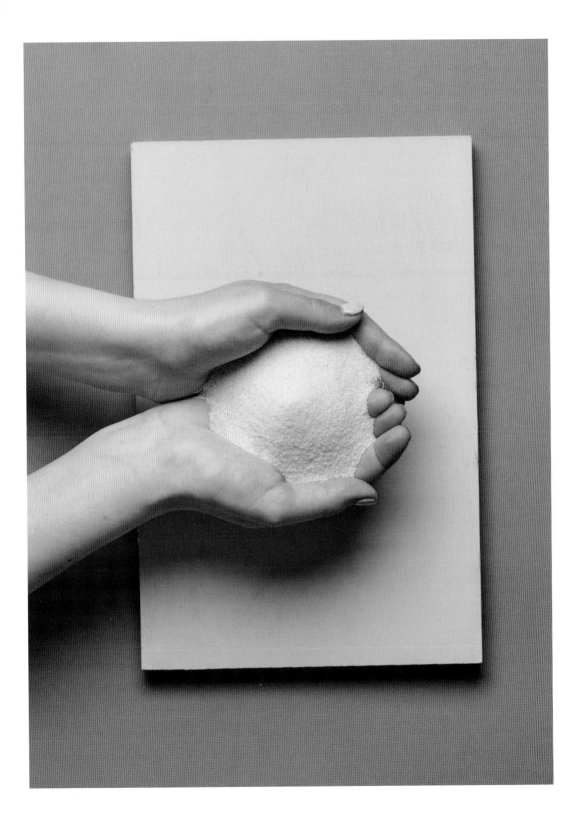

boob tube

20g beeswax
40ml avocado oil
40ml sweet almond oil
5ml carrot seed essential
   oil
5 drops pomegranate
   seed oil

MAKES:
100g

SHELF LIFE:
6 months in an airtight
container. Apply with clean
hands!

HELPFUL HINT:
This also works well as a lip
balm.

The skin on the chest is extremely fragile and, regardless of size, overexposure to the sun can result in the bust sagging and wrinkling much sooner than we'd all hope. This isn't helped if you're well endowed in that area; gravity does its work and the bouncy, no-bra days of your teens are well and truly over. We've put together a really powerful little number that will nourish that delicate skin and help to improve the appearance of those wrinkles. We're using both almond and avocado oils, which are high in potassium, proteins and vitamin A. This will penetrate the skin and help to replace elasticity and suppleness. We've also added carrot seed essential oil, which is renowned for helping improve the appearance of ageing skin, as well as beeswax which forms a protective layer over the top of skin to avoid damage from the elements. This also gives our Boob Tube a lovely, thick balm-like texture. Finally, the pomegranate seed oil makes this baby smell delightful!

1 Melt the beeswax in a bain-marie.
2 In a separate bowl, combine all the oils.
3 Mix the melted beeswax into the oils and stir well.
4 Store in an airtight jar and apply daily.

belly balm

15g shea butter

10g cocoa butter

20g coconut oil

5 drops lavender essential
oil

5 drops helichrysum
essential oil

5g beeswax

MAKES:
50g

SHELF LIFE:
6 months in an airtight
container. Apply with clean
hands!

HELPFUL HINT:
If you'd like a slightly
creamier texture then you
can experiment with the
amount of coconut oil you
use, or even add a liquid
carrier oil.

Stretch marks are one of those things – much like spots or cellulite – that we get asked about a lot. Niggly little things they are, caused when the skin both stretches and shrinks, and extremely hard to get rid of, not that you need to. They're formed in the dermis (the middle layer of the skin) so to be able to help improve their appearance, we have to find ingredients that can penetrate the skin and are rich enough to replace the elasticity that the skin has lost due to stretching. While it's difficult to completely get rid of stretch marks, what we plan to do is improve the quality of the skin and reduce redness to help improve their appearance. The combination of butters and beeswax really help this; they are moisturising, rich and create a seal that ultimately increases the suppleness of skin. Lavender has powerful healing qualities, whilst helichrysum, a powerfully healing essential oil, is widely used for cell renewal and skin rejuvenation.

---

1 Gently melt the butters in a bain-marie. Add the coconut oil and take off the heat.
2 Once slightly cooler, add the essential oils.
3 While the mixture is cooling melt the beeswax in a separate bowl using a bain-marie.
4 Combine the two mixtures and stir well.
5 Decant into a jar and allow to cool and harden.

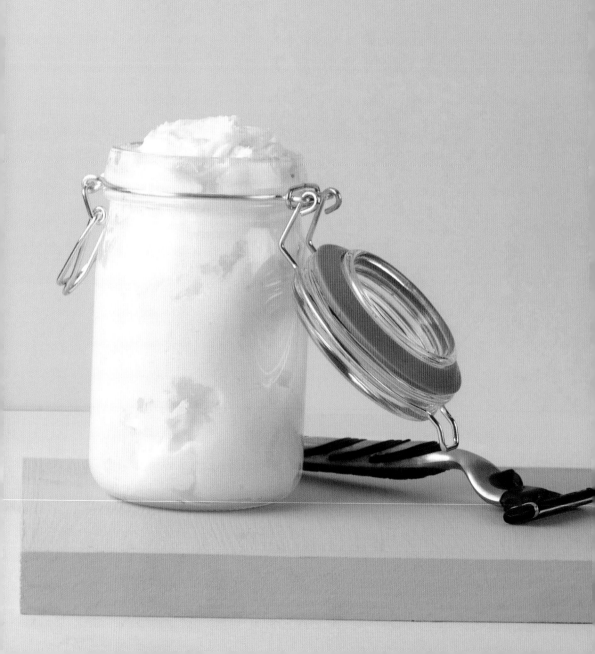

shave the day

20g coconut oil
10g mango butter
10g castor oil
**10ml Dr Bronner's Castile
Soap**

MAKES:
50g

SHELF LIFE:
6 months in an airtight
container.

HELPFUL HINT:
Jojoba oil also works really
nicely in this – either add to
the current mixture or swap
with the castor oil.

Getting our paws on a good shaving cream did make us wonder how we had survived without one for so long? Shaving creams help stop any friction between the blade and your skin, in turn reducing the risk of irritation and redness. Shaving puts a fair amount of stress on the skin and it can be dehydrating, leaving pores exposed to reactions and infections. So we've put together our most nourishing combination of oils and butters to ensure that you get a super-close shave and the skin left behind is supple and soft. Mango butter is highly underrated; it's incredibly high in vitamins A, C and E, which help to keep the skin strong and fight any infection from shaving. Castor oil is antibacterial as well a moisturising and will leave behind a gorgeous shine. The addition of Dr Bronner's helps to get that amazing foam texture that your high-street brands have, without resorting to harsh synthetics.

---

1 Melt the coconut oil and mango butter in a bain-marie.
2 Add the castor oil and stir well.
3 Place in the fridge and allow to cool until almost solid.
4 Finally add the Dr Bronner's to the mixture and whip with an electric whisk to achieve the foam texture. This should take a few minutes.
5 Decant into a pump or foam container.

say no to ingrowns

5ml boiled water
2 drops salicylic acid
10g honey

MAKES:
15ml

SHELF LIFE:
If kept in the fridge,
use within 1 week.
Alternatively, you can add
1 per cent preservative to
last up to 6 months.

HELPFUL HINT:
Keep the area well
moisturised to avoid
further ingrowns.

Godammit, those ingrown hairs are a right pain – often literally. Most people suffer from them at some point and they can be sore, unsightly and sometimes even embarrassing. Caused by the hair follicle curving round and quite literally growing in on itself, it's hard to prevent them if you're a regular shaver or waxer. This is very simple but hugely effective. Once you've bought the ingredients you can make it up as and when you need it. The golden ingredient here is salicylic acid. This stuff is an incredibly powerful acid and the natural option we use is extracted from the bark of the willow tree. It has powerful anti-inflammatory and antimicrobial properties, helps to unclog pores and exfoliate the affected area. Honey is incredibly antibacterial so will help fight any further infection, while also soothing the skin and replacing any lost moisture. It almost softens the power of the salicylic acid. This can be used all over: bikini line, legs, underarms… You name it, we've waxed it.

---

1 Dissolve the salicylic acid in the water. Stir well to ensure it's evenly distributed.
2 Stir in the honey and apply to the affected area. Allow to sit for up to 10 minutes before rinsing well.

bruise-you-lose balm

55ml jojoba oil
10g dried arnica herbs
35g beeswax
10 drops lavender
   essential oil

MAKES:
100g

SHELF LIFE:
6 months in an airtight container. Apply with clean hands!

HELPFUL HINT:
You can make up larger quantities of your infusion at one time and store in an airtight bottle. You can include other herbs, too; as long as they are dried and not fresh, the mixture will keep for up to 6 months. We love adding dried mint to the mix.

We are MEGA clumsy here at CBCo. Neither of us has been blessed with great coordination, despite being pretty active. This means that we're rarely seen without some sort of bruising, often the result of tumbling at the gym, tripping during a boxing session or even falling out of a handstand and into a bin (classic Dominika). We designed this number to help speed up the healing of our bumps and we store it in neat little pots that we can carry around in our handbags. The key here is, of course, arnica – an incredibly powerful herb that works wonders when it comes to healing sprains, strains and bruises. We've infused it in jojoba oil that has great anti-inflammatory properties, then added beeswax so that it takes on a balm-like texture. Finally, lavender is great at calming and soothing both the body and the mind, so that should help to ease the embarrassment of the latest topple.

1 Firstly you'll need to make an infusion out of your jojoba oil and arnica. Gently heat the jojoba oil in a bain-marie and add the arnica. Place a lid on the mixture and allow to very gently heat for 3–4 hours. You'll notice that the oil becomes darker and will eventually begin to smell like the arnica. At that stage you can remove it from the heat. Strain the herbs from the mixture.
2 In a separate bowl, heat the beeswax in a bain-marie until liquid, then add the lavender. Slowly add the infusion to the wax mixture, stirring thoroughly.
3 Decant into a balm container and place in the fridge to cool and harden. Use as and when needed but do not use on open wounds.

neat little deo bars

50g coconut oil

20g shea butter

10g arrowroot powder

10g bicarbonate of soda

5 drops peppermint
essential oil

5 drops tea tree essential
oil

5 drops frankincense
essential oil

10g beeswax

MAKES:
100g

SHELF LIFE:
6 months; store in an airtight
container.

HELPFUL HINT:
We like the convenience of
having these in handy little
bars. However, if you prefer
a balm texture that you can
apply with your fingers, omit
the beeswax from the recipe
and store in a jar instead.

We get asked a lot about natural deodorant, mainly because there are many stories flying around about parabens in store-bought deodorants being found in the tissues of breast cancers. Whether true or not, there's no doubt that your average high-street deo is high in synthetic chemicals and metals that we'd prefer to keep away from our boobs, thank you very much. Having said that, making the switch to natural is often a process that people find challenging and that's mainly because you have to come to terms with the fact that a natural antiperspirant doesn't exist: it's not natural to not sweat. Your body needs to sweat, it's its way of releasing toxins and waste from the body, and clogging up your glands to try to avoid this is not a healthy thing to do. Natural deodorants will just help to stop that sweat being stinky. We love these handy little bars as they're extremely moisturising for the delicate underarm area (that'll be the coconut oil and shea butter), with antibacterial properties from the arrowroot and essential oils. This will help stop bacteria growing and smelly odours occurring. Bicarbonate of soda helps absorb patches of wet while also balancing out the skin's pH, where an imbalance may lead to odour. Our powerful combination of essential oils should keep you smelling super-fresh all day.

---

1 Melt the coconut oil and shea butter in a bain-marie.
2 Stir in the arrowroot, bicarbonate of soda and essential oils.
3 In a separate bowl, heat in the beeswax in a bain-marie.
4 Once liquid, slowly add to the coconut oil mixture and stir well.
5 Decant into a silicon muffin tray; we're using a mould roughly
3 × 3cm, and place in the fridge to cool until solid.
6 Store the bars in a jar in the fridge and use by gently rubbing in
with a couple of swipes.

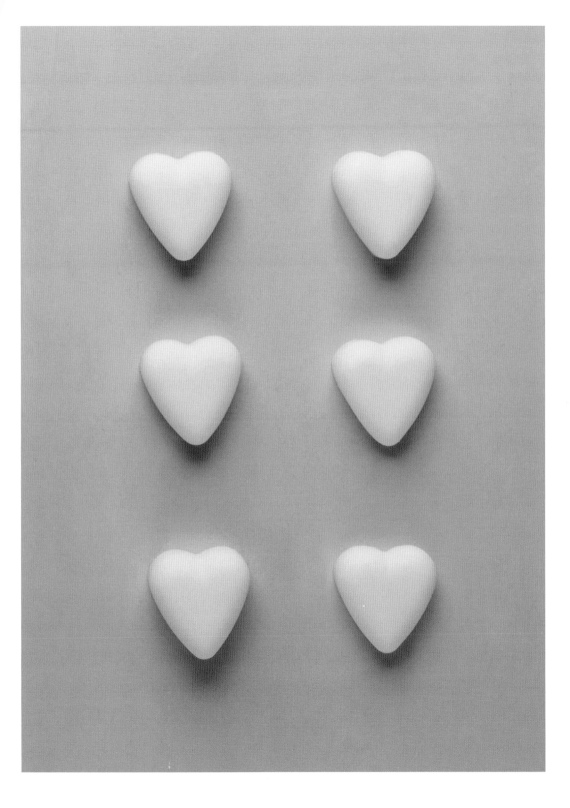

freshen up

5 drops tangerine
   essential oil
5ml vegetable glycerine
50ml rose hydrosol
45ml orange blossom
   hydrosol

_____

MAKES:
100ml

SHELF LIFE:
3 months if using pre-
preserved floral waters; if not
store in the fridge and use
within 1 week.

HELPFUL HINT:
A combo of lavender and
chamomile water is another
alternative – ultra soothing!

Floral waters are a great way to add scent to a recipe while also benefiting from the properties of the plant itself. We love using this little number as a bit of a multi-purpose freshener; you can spritz it all over after a long day in the sun as a way to cool and nourish the skin, or alternatively you can use it as a body spray or even a deodorant. The combination of rose and orange blossom has a light, floral scent that's in no way overpowering. Rosewater also has great antibacterial properties, which means it's good to freshen up your pits after a particularly sweaty day. We wanted to enhance the citrus smell in this one by using an essential oil but as we mentioned earlier on, oil and water don't mix. We've therefore included glycerine; it doesn't completely break the tangerine oil down but it disperses it enough to be safe to use on the skin. Please note: many citrus oils can be phototoxic, which means they can't be used in the sun. Tangerine oil is not phototoxic, so please ensure you don't swap it for any other citrus alternative.

_____

1 Add the tangerine oil to the glycerine and stir well to ensure it is evenly distributed.
2 Combine the waters and add to the glycerine mixture.
3 Decant into a spray mist bottle and shake well before each use.

nailed it

45ml sweet almond oil

5 drops pomegranate seed oil

2 drops myrrh essential oil

2 drops peppermint essential oil

2 drops rosemary essential oil

5g beeswax

MAKES:
50ml

SHELF LIFE:
6 months in an airtight container.

HELPFUL HINT:
This is also fabulous for toenails, cracked heels, dry elbows or knees, or even for rubbing into the scalp to promote hair growth.

We spent years getting harsh Shellac and Gelish manicures on a bi-weekly basis and unfortunately it had a bit of an effect on our nails, leaving them dry, brittle and pretty hard to grow. Switching to non-toxic nail polishes has helped a lot, but we still find our nails have the tendency to be pretty soft. We designed this nail oil to help encourage growth and to repair the nail bed, cuticle and surrounding skin. Myrrh essential oil has often been used in medicine as it has powerful healing properties, is anti-inflammatory and can help soothe irritated skin. The combination of peppermint and rosemary essential oils is a great circulatory stimulant, helping blood flow and in turn promoting the growth of the skin and nails. We've chosen sweet almond as our carrier as its naturally high vitamin E content will help repair broken skin and deeply moisturise. This one has a pretty powerful smell but just think of all the goodness it'll bring to your talons!

---

1 Add the essential oils to the carrier oils and stir well.

2 Melt the beeswax in a bain-marie and mix in with the oils.

3 Decant into a jar and use as often as needed.

customisable hand washes

200ml Dr Bronner's Castile Soap
Up to 20 drops of a combination of essential oils (see opposite for our faves)

MAKES:
200ml

SHELF LIFE:
6 months in an airtight container.

HELPFUL HINT:
You can throw in a splash of a carrier oil such as jojoba for a moisture injection.

This is a super-simple recipe that gives you the chance to get a little creative, because who said that hand washing couldn't be fun? Not us. The base for this one is our trusty Dr Bronner's, a wonderfully cleansing liquid soap. While you can buy his soaps ready flavoured, we like to add our own stamp on things, particularly when it comes to scent. So we're using the neutral soap and throwing in our own essential oils! This is a great and very basic way to explore the properties and fragrance of different oils. Why not try a combination of three oils to begin with? Tea tree, lemongrass and lavender for an antibacterial winner? Frankincense, helichrysum and rose for an anti-ageing superstar? Or just keep it plain and simple with geranium, tangerine or carrot seed? Why not create one for each room in the house? The choices are endless and allow you to do some practical research and develop your essential oil knowledge, without being a super-complex and intimidating recipe.

1 Combine the Dr Bronner's with the essential oils and stir well.
2 Store in a pump-cap bottle.

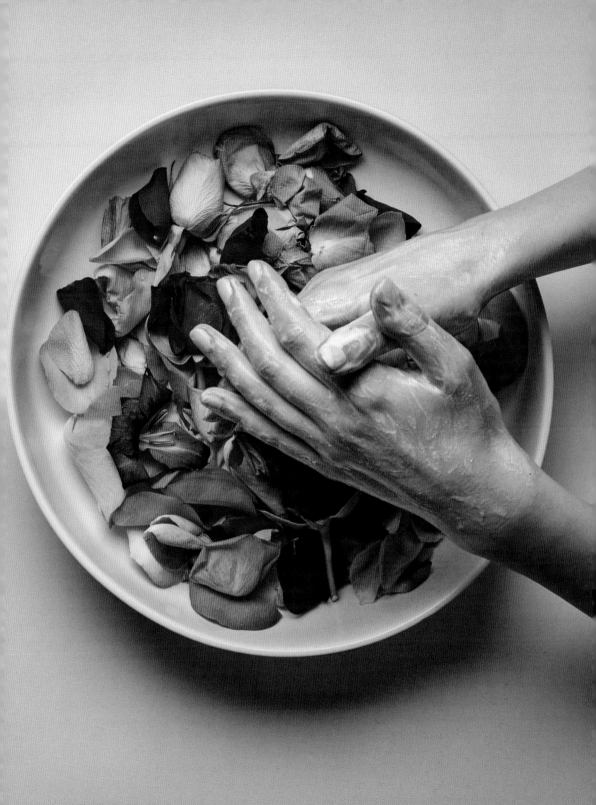

Friends don't let friends
have bad eyebrows.

hair

nutty shampoo

50ml distilled water, boiled
a handful of broken soap nuts
5ml vegetable glycerine

MAKES:
50ml

SHELF LIFE:
1 week in the fridge if left unpreserved. Add a water-soluble preservative to extend the shelf life to 6 months.

HELPFUL HINT:
You can customise this shampoo by adding essential oils or natural proteins like rice protein, which will strengthen your locks.

Soap nuts are becoming an increasingly attractive and eco-friendly way of washing your clothes. This chemical-free technique of care is incredibly appealing for people trying to lead clean lifestyles. Also known as Indian Soap Nuts, they grow on trees and are a source of saponin, a natural surfactant (for more on surfactants see p. 27) that cleans and freshens. The nuts can also be used to create a super-easy and effective shampoo. The shampoo foams but doesn't create a lather like normal shampoo; but rest assured, it is giving your hair a good clean!

---

1 Pour the boiled distilled water onto the nuts in a bowl.
2 Leave to soak for 12 hours.
3 Drain the water from the soap nuts into a bowl (the water is the stuff you need, not the nuts).
4 Throw away the soap nuts.
5 Add the glycerine to the soap nut water.
6 Decant into a clear bottle.

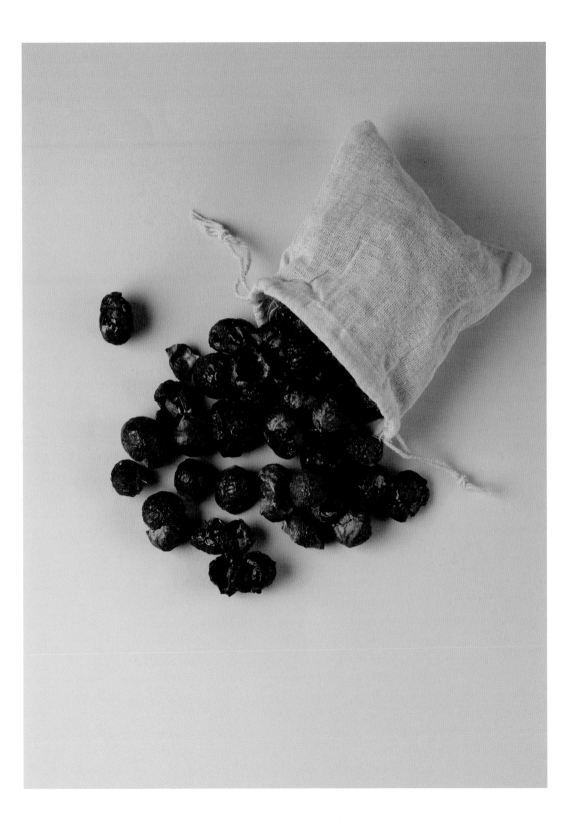

rapunzel's serum

20ml grapeseed oil
20ml avocado oil
10ml castor oil
2 drops rosemary extract
2 drops lavender
  essential oil

MAKES:
50ml

SHELF LIFE:
6 months.

HELPFUL HINT:
Rosemary extract is an antioxidant like vitamin E, so it slows down the rancidity of the oils. We're using it here because rosemary is also beneficial for maintaining healthy hair.

This hair serum is designed to promote healthy hair growth by toning the scalp and conditioning the hair root. Grapeseed oil is a fab addition to any hair serum; rich in vitamin E and linoleic acid, it strengthens and repairs damaged locks. Avocado is highly nourishing for the hair, with humectant properties that lock in moisture, conditioning and strengthening the strands. Castor oil is rich in ricinoleic acid and omega-6 essential fatty acids, which encourage hair growth and balance the scalp's pH. Rosemary and lavender are beneficial for the scalp; they are powerful stimulants encouraging blood circulation, working against inflammation that causes dandruff and flaking, fostering new hair growth. They also smell like a garden – ahhh.

---

1 Blend the carrier oils.
2 Add the rosemary extract and lavender essential oil.
3 Decant into a pump bottle.

lazy-girls' shampoo

45g arrowroot powder
5g bicarbonate of soda
5 drops lavender
   essential oil

MAKES:
50g

SHELF LIFE:
6 months if stored in an airtight container. Keep fingers out and make sure to shake well before every use.

HELPFUL HINT:
Arrowroot powder can also be used as a make-up setter or as a refresher throughout the day to absorb excess oil.

The theory behind dry shampoos is that they put an oil-absorbing substance on the roots of your hair to suck up the oils and have you looking fine and fresh. We're not just being lazy, OK? It's actually better to wash your hair less, so use this when you're trying to lengthen out those long stints between washes. Arrowroot is a natural powdered root starch that is lightweight and white in colour. If you are dark-haired, you could add cocoa powder to darken the shade and avoid the granny-grey look you can get on the five-day stretches. A make-up brush is a fab way to apply dry shampoo, but make sure you wash it regularly. If you can't find arrowroot, cornflour will also do.

1 Combine the three ingredients in a bowl. Mix well and evenly.
2 Decant into a container; a salt shaker isn't a bad idea, but you could also use a make-up pot and brush to dab it on.
3 Use on the hair root instead of washing.

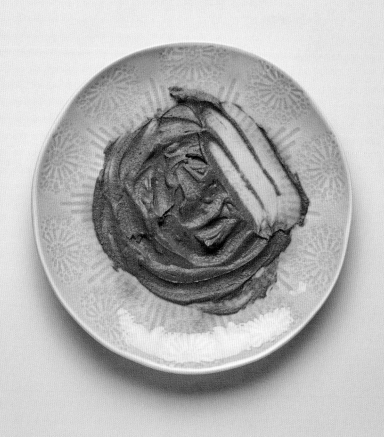

moroccan hair wash

3 tablespoons rhassoul clay
3 tablespoons water

MAKES:
50g

SHELF LIFE:
One-time use; use immediately.

HELPFUL HINT:
This can get messy so be sure to rinse the shower post-use!

It's a strange sensation washing your hair with clay and not shampoo, but go on, we dare you to give it a try and we won't say we told you so when your hair looks phenomenal! Rhassoul clay is harvested in Morocco and it is used as a shampoo or mild soap because of its exceptional ability to bind fat and carry water. Unlike shampoos and soaps, rhassoul contains no surfactants and cleans by absorbing impurities and fat. It extracts fat from the skin and hair while not irritating the sebaceous glands, like many shampoos that contain synthetic surfactants. If you're trying out the no-shampoo method (affectionately known as the no-poo method – don't be afraid to Google that) then this one's for you!

---

1 Mix the clay and water together to form a runny paste.
2 Dip the ends into the mud wash and then pour the rest over the roots.
3 Leave to sit for 5 minutes and then follow up with an alkalising Apple Cider Vinegar Rinse (p. 101).

going nuts for nutter

20ml argan oil
30ml carrier oil of your
   choice
1 drop vitamin E oil

MAKES:
50ml

SHELF LIFE:
6 months, but keep wet
fingers out if you're keeping
it in the shower.

HELPFUL HINT:
This can be used on the tips
of dry hair (one pump), on
wet, freshly washed hair (two
pumps), or as an overnight
treatment before you wash
your hair (three pumps).

Hair serums are the way to go when prepping your hair pre- or post-shower. We love them because they can be used on dry hair as a post-wash styling serum with one squirt or a heavier treatment on wet hair. When we started our DIY journey, we were desperate to replace our so-called 'argan' hair oils, which didn't contain much argan at all. Nutter has been flying off the shelves ever since and so we had to include it here. We've also provided tons of customising options; we know all too well that everyone's hair is different and one woman's conditioner is another's greasy nightmare. There are a myriad carrier oils that hold beneficial properties for the hair and using argan oil as your base, we encourage you to find other oils that your hair loves and drinks up. Or if you want to use our tried and tested formula of sweet almond and macadamia nut oil with a hint of geranium, that's golden too. Either way, your hair is going to look a million bucks.

---

1 Blend the argan oil with your carrier oil.
2 Add your essential oil and vitamin E oil.
3 Decant into a pump bottle.

Carrier Oil: Avocado (dry), castor (frizzy), coconut (damaged), jojoba (oily), sesame (curly), hemp seed (thin)… these are all delicious for your hair. Refer to Carrier Oils 101 (p. 22) for further inspiration.

Optional: Five drops of your essential oil of choice. You can choose both for scent and for healing properties. Refer to Essential Oils 101 (p. 26) for further inspiration.

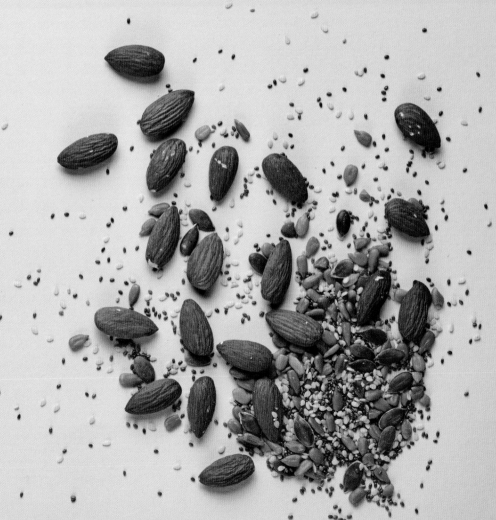

his beard gear

10ml argan oil
10ml sweet almond oil
10ml fractionated
   coconut oil
1 drop rosemary
   antioxidant
1 drop cedarwood
   essential oil

Beard oil is the ultimate male accessory. The downside to the hipster beard being suuhhh trendy is that they are usually scratchy, spindly and not adequately conditioned for our soft faces. Treat the bearded male in your life to a masculine-scented beard oil, sneakily concocted with tendril-soothing oils that will stop your Movember fear in its tracks. The oils will condition, moisturise and strengthen the hair and the rosemary and cedarwood provide the manly scent.

MAKES:
30ml

SHELF LIFE:
6 months in an airless pump bottle.

HELPFUL HINT:
Patchouli, rosemary or clove essential oil are also good for that masculine scent.

1 Blend the carrier oils.
2 Add the rosemary antioxidant and cedarwood essential oil.
3 Decant into a bottle.

dem curlz styling cream

35g shea butter
15g beeswax
35g coconut oil
15ml castor oil
5 drops tangerine
   essential oil

_____

MAKES:
100g

SHELF LIFE:
6 months in an airtight
container.

HELPFUL HINT:
For finer curls, use less
beeswax and more coconut
oil. For coarser curls, up the
beeswax and use slightly
less coconut oil.

This is our version of a curly-haired girl's styling cream. Typical slippery silicone serums don't do beautiful curls justice and leaves them coated in plastic, so we've made something clean and with more muscle. We want to moisturise deeply but we don't want to leave the hair too weighed down or sticky. Having said that, the cream needs to be heavy enough to smooth flyaways. We present your new BFF: a customisable crème to help you keep your curls healthy, bouncy and alive. Coconut oil is super-nourishing for the hair; it is comprised of smaller medium-chain fatty acids, so it penetrates the hair more deeply than other oils. Shea and beeswax gives the cream its creamy consistency, while also protecting the hair against damage and pollution. Castor oil is all about the shine but also smoothes and controls frizz.

_____

1 Melt the butter and beeswax together in a bain-marie.
2 Stir in the coconut and castor oils.
3 Once cooled, stir in your tangerine oil.
4 Decant into a jar or squeezy tube.

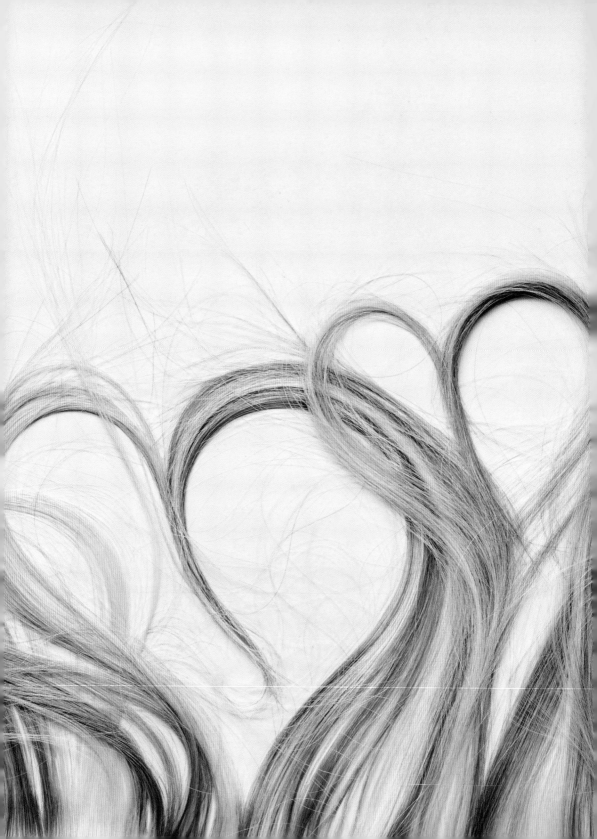

beach waves

5g Epsom salts
3g pink Himalayan salt
20ml boiled water
2 drops vegetable glycerine
4 drops lavender essential oil

Salt sprays were inspired by the tousled locks often found on bronzed beach lovers. The idea is that you can recreate that 'don't mind me, I've just been surfing' look, even if a beach is or feels even further away than Mars. Salt creates amazing texture in the hair, and Epsom salts are less drying than sea salt. The glycerine is added to make sure your new beach waves set and don't fall out. There's something magical about the smell of lavender and salt, not to mention how great lavender is for the locks. Surf's up!

MAKES:
30ml

SHELF LIFE:
1 week in the fridge if unpreserved. Add a water-soluble preservative to extend the shelf life to 6 months.

HELPFUL HINT:
You can add 5ml alcohol, for example, vodka, to preserve this product which will extend the shelf life to 6 months. But it can be drying for the hair over time so be sure to follow up with a wash with a nourishing hair treatment like Banana Head (p. 105).

1 Dissolve the salts in the boiled water.
2 Wait until cool, then add the glycerine and essential oil.
3 Shake well before use.

dry as the sahara

**40ml Dr Bronner's Castile
 Soap**
5ml sweet almond oil
5ml vegetable glycerine
**5 drops lemon essential
 oil**

Dr Bronner's provides the perfect base to make a DIY shampoo
– it's naturally foaming, mild and also a foundation ingredient,
meaning you can customise it to suit your hair type. For this
dry-hair shampoo, we've added glycerine to lock in moisture
and sweet almond oil for conditioning; the oil absorbs quickly
and won't weigh down dry, thin hair. Lemon cleanses deeply,
promotes shine and nourishes the hair follicle.

MAKES:
50ml

SHELF LIFE:
6 months in an airless pump
container.

1 Combine the Dr Bronner's with the sweet almond oil and glycerine.
2 Stir in the essential oil.
3 Decant into a pump bottle.

HELPFUL HINT:
Follow up with our Apple
Cider Vinegar Rinse (p. 101)
if the scalp feels itchy; Dr
Bronner's is quite alkaline
and can throw the scalp
pH off balance.

shine serum

15ml argan oil
15ml avocado oil
15ml olive oil
5ml pomegranate seed oil
5 drops grapefruit
    essential oil
1 drop rosemary
    antioxidant

For our serum, four moisturising oils join forces to give your hair serious shine. Argan is commonly referred to in Morocco as liquid gold and it is extremely rich in beneficial nutrients for the hair, like vitamin E and fatty acids. Avocado and olive oils are great moisturisers, repairing dry and damaged hair, but they are also lightweight and absorb quickly. Pomegranate seed oil is rich in punicic acid, which is revitalising, leaving hair looking thick and shiny. It's also a great protector against chemicals and other environmental damage that cause free radicals. Grapefruit gives the serum an enticing scent but it will also keep you frizz-free.

MAKES:
50ml

SHELF LIFE:
6 months in an airtight container.

1 Blend the carrier oils.
2 Add the essential oil and antioxidant.
3 Decant into a dark bottle.

HELPFUL HINT:
This is a rich serum, so you only need a small squirt on dry hair to reap the benefits.

colour brightener

30ml sweet almond oil
5 drops essential oil
   of your choice (see
   opposite for our faves)

MAKES:
30ml

SHELF LIFE:
6 months in an airtight
pump container.

HELPFUL HINT:
For thicker hair, you could
use argan or macadamia
nut oils.

While essential oils cannot alter the colour of your hair, certain ones can enhance colour and protect from colouring damage. Chamomile brightens and enhances blondes, sage is great for darker tones and carrot seed oil works wonders for ravishing reds. Sweet almond oil is incredibly light and easily absorbed so it provides the perfect base for your colour protector. Use as a daily serum post washing for optimum benefits.

---

1 Blend the oil and essential oil.
2 Decant into a dark bottle.

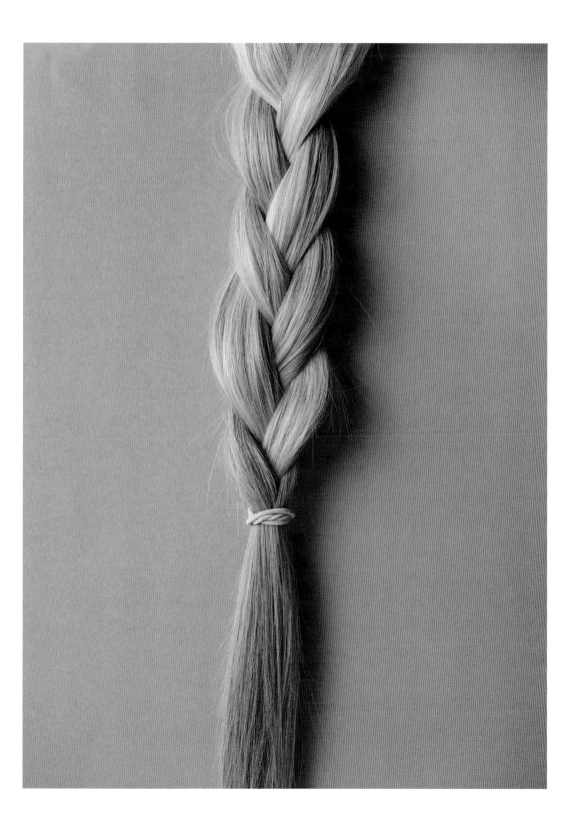

hair milk mask

20g coconut oil
5ml jojoba oil
5ml argan oil
20ml coconut milk

MAKES:
50ml

SHELF LIFE:
1 week in the fridge.

HELPFUL HINT:
You can leave out the coconut milk until you want to make a mask, and then you have a good hair serum to use in between.

This mask is perfect as a pre-shampoo treat, super-moisturising and repairing for the hair. Applying coconut milk directly to the scalp is beneficial for healthy hair growth, as it is rich in niacin and folate, stimulating blood circulation. Jojoba is an excellent treatment for dry scalps as it regulates sebum production and helps to balance the scalp's pH. Coconut and argan are super hair oils, but you can always substitute olive, macadamia nut, sweet almond or avocado if you prefer these for your hair.

---

1 Blend the oils.
2 Stir in the coconut milk.
3 Decant into an airtight container.
4 Apply to dry, dirty hair for 10 minutes before shampooing.

babassu shampoo cubes

25ml babassu oil
25g coconut oil
5 drops grapefruit
essential oil

MAKES:
10 cubes

SHELF LIFE:
6 months if stored in an
airtight container or in the
fridge.

HELPFUL HINT:
Ice-cube trays are the
perfect size for one use.

Babassu is a great oil to get to know on your DIY journey. It's often compared to coconut oil as they have similar chemical structures: high in lauric acid, emollient, high levels of vitamin E and deeply penetrating. Babassu is also a natural surfactant, meaning that it foams when heated. Similar to coconut oil, it solidifies at cooler temperatures, making the duo the perfect consistency for shampoo bars. Grapefruit and coconut oil also make a killer combo for the senses. You'll need a setting tray for this one!

---

1 Melt the babassu and coconut oils in a bain-marie and stir vigorously.
2 Stir in the essential oil when cool and decant into a mould.
3 Leave to set and keep somewhere cool, or in the fridge, otherwise they will melt.

summer serum

20ml argan oil
15ml macadamia nut oil
   or sweet almond oil
10ml monoi oil
5ml vegetable glycerine
1 drop vitamin E oil

This serum is perfect for the warmer and humid summer months; it's light and will be absorbed without leaving a greasy residue on your tender locks. Glycerine is added to provide texture and styling to the serum, keeping hair in place and summer frizz at bay. Monoi oil is a super hair oil from Polynesia; it helps with the general hair condition, repairing dry and damaged hair, but also smells like a tropical island. When we're on holiday it looks a little like this: cocktail to the right, serum to left.

MAKES:
50ml

SHELF LIFE:
6 months in an airtight container.

1 Blend the oils and glycerine.
2 Add the vitamin E.
3 Decant into a pump bottle.

HELPFUL HINT:
You could use squalane or castor oil instead of glycerine.

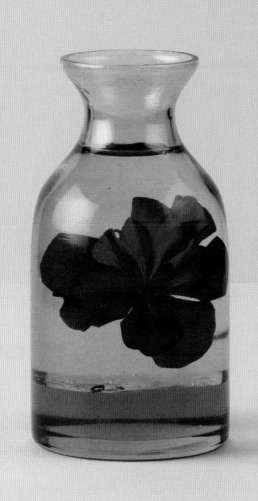

scalp scrub

10ml olive oil
30ml Dr Bronner's Castile Soap
10g pink Himalayan sea salt

MAKES:
50g

SHELF LIFE:
3 months in an airtight container. Use a scoop to reduce the introduction of water into the product.

HELPFUL HINT:
Use only once a month as overuse can be quite drying on the hair.

We're used to using scrubs on our bodies and faces to slough away dead skin cells, but the same practice can be applied to hair. This purifying salt scrub removes any dry flakes or dandruff, dissolves excess product residue, removes dust and pollution build-up and also gives a boost of volume. The olive oil will coat the hair, providing moisture and protection against damage. Use instead of a shampoo and follow up with a conditioner or hair treatment.

---

1 Mix the olive oil and Dr Bronner's liquid soap.
2 Stir in the sea salt.
3 Decant into a container and use once a month, as above.

nettle thickening spray

45ml nettle hydrosol
5g maca root liquid extract

MAKES:
50ml

SHELF LIFE:
3 months if using pre-preserved hydrosol.

HELPFUL HINT:
Maca root powder can work if you're in a pinch, but the liquid extract blends better.

Nettle is an absolute dream for thin hair: fortifying, mineralising and balancing, rich in proteins and high in natural silica. It is a great thickener and perfect for use as a post-shampoo toner. Maca has been used in traditional therapies to stimulate hair growth, by promoting keratinocytes to the hair bulbs. Keratinocytes are the cells which produce keratin, a protein that protects the hair from damage and stress. Keratin also improves hair viscosity, by making it tougher and thicker. This one's a real treat for tired, thin tresses.

---

1 Blend the hydrosol and maca.
2 Decant into a spray bottle.
3 Shake well before use.
4 Apply on dry hair as needed.

after eight shampoo cubes

50ml coconut milk
25ml aloe vera gel
**10 drops peppermint
   essential oil**

MAKES:
20 cubes

SHELF LIFE:
6 months if frozen; 2 days
once defrosted.

HELPFUL HINT:
You can add a natural
foamer like babassu if you
want the shampoo to foam
slightly.

Coconut milk, like coconut oil, is high in essential fatty acids, which will moisturise hair making it soft, silky and easy to handle. Those same properties are also great for dry scalps too. Aloe vera is not widely recognised as a hair treatment but it is an effective addition; it contains proteolytic enzymes, which help to repair skin cells on the scalp and is also high in amino acids, which can promote strength and shine. Peppermint is perfect for a dry scalp; it sooths dry and itchy skin and helps prevent dandruff. It balances the scalp's sebum production without making it over active.

---

1 Blend the coconut milk and aloe vera until you have a smooth, runny paste.
2 Add the essential oil.
3 Decant into ice-cube trays and freeze.
4 Defrost each cube before use.

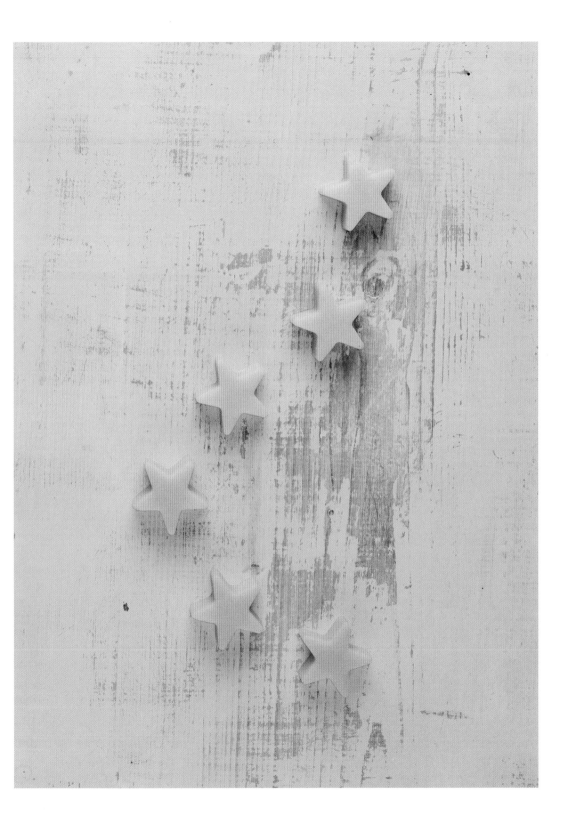

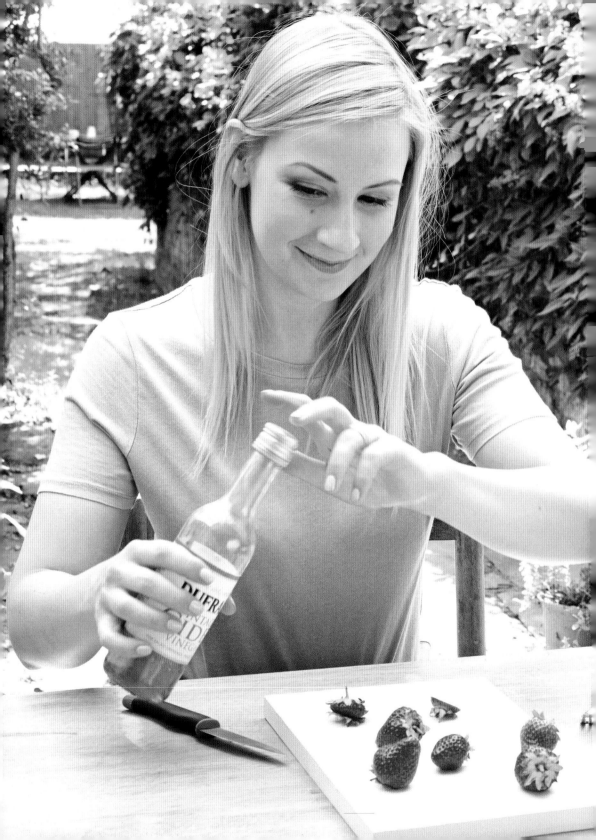

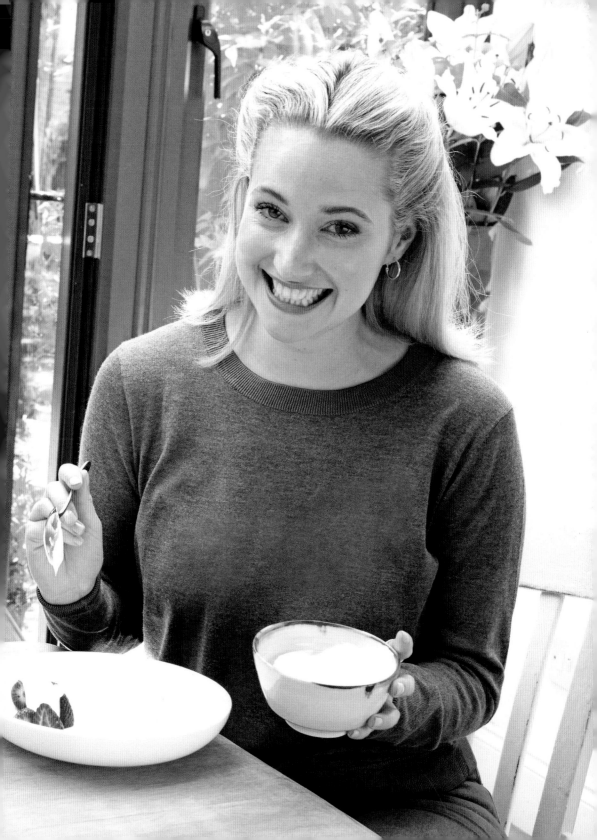

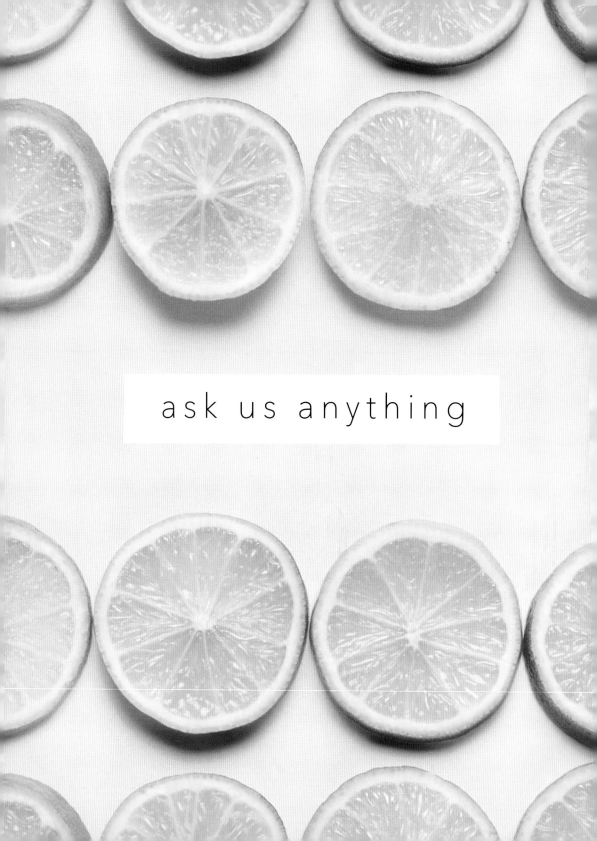

ask us anything

Will my homemade products work as well as shop-bought alternatives?

Yup. DIY beauty means you have total control over what goes into your products. You're using high quantities of the best ingredients and getting rid of any pointless fillers that have no benefit. Not only is this better for your health but you'll find your homemade goodies make for healthier-looking skin and hair too. It's win-win.

Are these ingredients really expensive?

Absolutely not. If you don't already have them in your kitchen, chances are they are found on your local supermarket shelves or on Amazon. Buy organic where possible; the price point is higher, but these ingredients haven't been exposed to potentially harmful chemicals and pesticides. If not, where possible, give them a really good wash before using them.

Where do I get all these ingredients from?

There were some interesting names in these recipes, right? Don't fear. We promise we wouldn't leave you up the creek without a paddle; we're absolute babes like that. At the time of writing, most of the ingredients can be found either on websites like Amazon or in your local supermarket or health-food store. The rest of the DIY beauty goodies can be found at wholesalers of natural cosmetics ingredients: in the UK try Aromantic, Gracefruit and Naturally Thinking.

I want to make a recipe but don't have one of the ingredients. Can I substitute something similar?

Sure! We wholeheartedly encourage you to get a little creative in the kitchen. The only exception is when dealing with essential oils. Don't forget the 1 per cent rule: ensure that your essential oils total no more than 1 per cent of the entire recipe quantity. You should also thoroughly research the properties of each essential oil before substituting one oil for another.

My recipe smells funky, what should I do?

Well, that depends on the level of funky. If you've used a blend of oils that comes off less floral and more swamp, you can use essential oils to mask the undesirable scents. Not all carrier oils are created equal and some do have rather unique smells. However, if your product smells off, or has any mould, then… Throw. It. Away. Immediately. Using mouldy products anywhere on your body is a health hazard and can have serious side effects.

Why is the shelf life of these products and natural beauty products so short?

There's something uncomfortably artificial to us about a face cream lasting three years. Would we expect to eat an apple that old and have all the nutrients still intact? Natural products are natural, so it's expected that they couldn't and shouldn't last as long as their synthetic counterparts. Active botanicals, clays, floral waters and all the other wonderful potent ingredients can be manipulated to last longer, but it usually involves destroying the natural synergies that we're including them for! The potency means we're using less, wasting less and ultimately only need smaller amounts to do the job. Your recipe needs to be used within 6 months…? Don't worry; you'll use it up and more!

I've seen loads of recipes on the Internet, can I make those?

There is a lot of great content on the Internet but there is also content written by amateurs who unknowingly publish unsafe recipes. By following our principles of clean beauty, you'll be sure that whatever you make remains safe and effective.

I'm buying oils that say pure; does this mean they are organic and natural?

We wish! But no, unfortunately not. The terms 'pure' and 'natural' have no legal classification in beauty, and many brands claim to be organic without the proper certification. Research your brands and buy from reputable and ethical companies. If a product's cheap, it's probably because it's of inferior quality. If it's claiming to be organic and you're paying a premium for this, look out for the Soil Association logo.

I don't have a preservative but I've added water to my product, what should I do?

Refrigerate and use it within a week. We don't want to sound like bores – we promise there's better ways to live on the edge – but don't risk using contaminated products on the skin. It's real, it hurts and it ain't going to make you look like a million bucks. We are taught that unpreserved food is the way to go: unfortunately in cosmetics, it's not. If it's got water, it needs a preservative or it will go off – and fast.

You've talked a lot about preservatives and water, I get it! It sounds hard, though, how do I incorporate a preservative into my products?

It's not that hard and really requires experimentation more than anything. The ideal preservative is 'broad spectrum', meaning that it kills off bacteria, mould, yeast and other fungi. There are some great natural broad-spectrum preservatives on the market that will adequately protect your products for normally up to a year. We love to use Preservative Eco, Liquid Leucidal or combo Sodium Benzoate/Potassium Sorbate.

Preservatives are normally added at 1 per cent and in the 'cool down' phase, i.e. the point where your product is cooling and not freshly heated. Also check your product pH using pH strips (which can be found on Amazon) before and after adding the preservative, as many become ineffective if your product is outside a particular measurement. There are also ingredients that can make your preservative ineffective, for example certain emulsifiers. The instructions on this, the pH range, the percentage and how to blend will be shared by the supplier of your preservative, so make sure to read the instructions and ask questions!

Keep reaching for the
stars, but please... get
a better deodorant.

index

index: ingredients

index: treatments

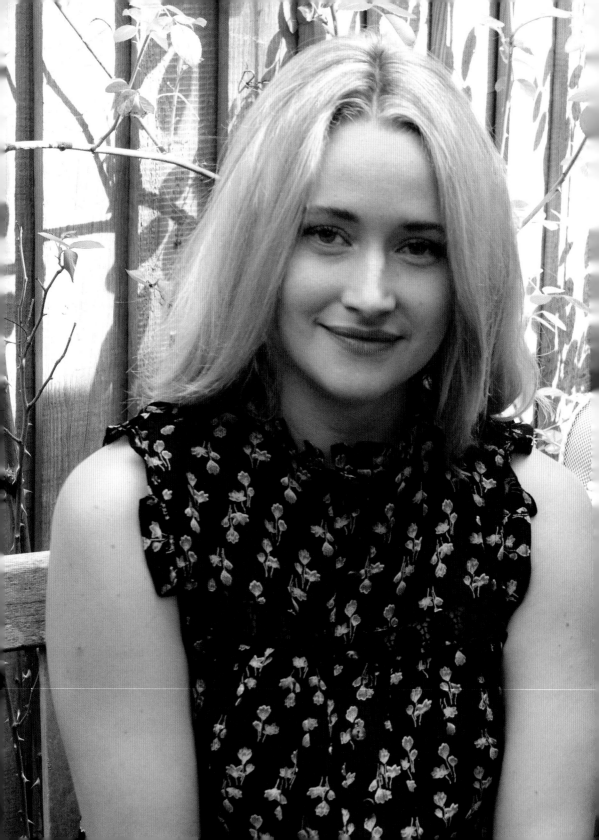

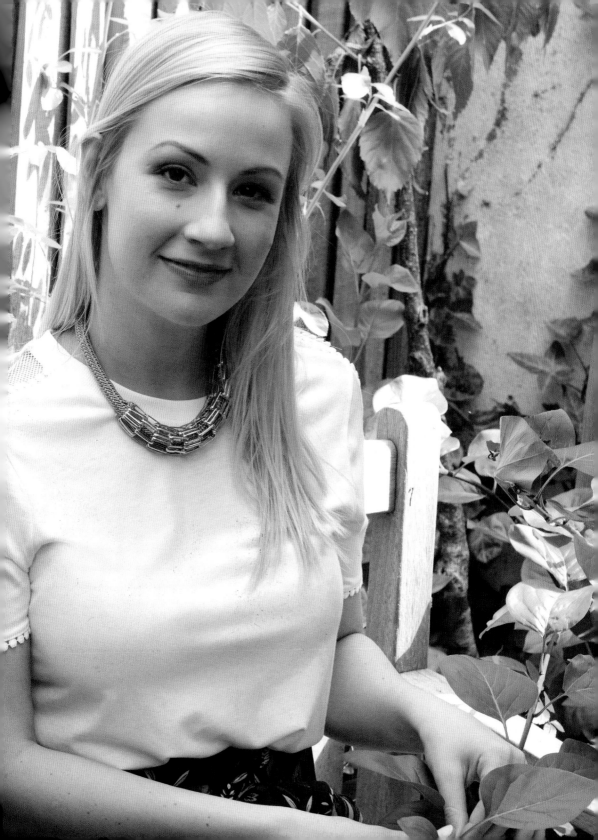

acknowledgements

Thank you to our agent Richard at Curtis Brown; who went out and passionately pitched the book when DIY body scrubs were probably not what he did in his spare time. To our wonderful Square Peg team: Susannah, Rowan, Naomi, who from day one got behind the idea of smothering themselves in coffee and avocado and are now converted clean beauties. Your belief and passion means so much to us. To Charlotte, who helped us bring our vision to life and didn't question when we started making heart shapes with hair. To Anna, for creating such a stunning book and Laura at Cuckoo PR, you're the best, we don't know what we'd do without you.

We are so lucky to be surrounded by friends and family who have supported us from day one. Thank you to our parents for encouraging us to follow our dreams and special shoutout to our wonderful mums for their endless advice, ideas and enthusiasm. To Nana, who regularly gives impromptu science lessons, is now a coffee scrub convert and who keeps a keen eye on CBCo goings on from the other side of the world; your support means so much. To Darcy, a little ray of sunshine who regularly makes us smile with her unfalteringly positive messages. Thank you to our men, who get up early on Sundays, ferry us around to all our events and pretend to be interested when we chat on about what oats can do for your skin: Luke, CBCo's very own facemask guinea pig and in-house practical joker and Sam, who hasn't blinked an eye at us using our house as everything from a lab, to storage facility, manufacturing premises and office. We honestly don't know where we'd be without you both.

Thank you to our biggest fans: Sophy, who's probably lost a ton of Facebook friends for the amount she shares about CBCo, Josh, who is unashamedly our number one Instagram fan and we're sure secretly makes all of our recipes on Friday nights, Lisa, who is always with us unwaveringly willing to help a hand or carry a box, and to Harriet, who will rave to anyone that mentions the word beauty and insists they try one of our magic potions. Thank you to everyone that we've worked with along the way, you've been instrumental in developing the brand into what it is today: Mel (miraculously manages to make us look less awkward in photos), Becky (helping us shape our brand's design since day one), James (what a website) and Adria, Sara, Lucie, Katie, Tabby, Mayah, Sabrina, Maria... you guys rock.

And above all, thank you to our clean beauty crew: everyone that has ever made our recipes, followed us on social, has come to a workshop or bought our products. We quite literally wouldn't be here without you and we hope you love the book!

1 3 5 7 9 10 8 6 4 2

Square Peg, an imprint of Vintage,
20 Vauxhall Bridge Road,
London SW1V 2SA

Square Peg is part of the Penguin Random House group of companies whose
addresses can be found at global.penguinrandomhouse.com.

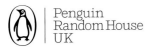

Penguin
Random House
UK

First published by Square Peg in 2017

www.vintage-books.co.uk

A CIP catalogue record for this book is available from the British Library

ISBN 9781910931455

Design by Anna Green at www.siulendesign.com
Photography by Charlotte Kibbles
Make up by Tabby Castro
Additional images: p. 11 © Melissa Gamvros;
p. 16-17, 19, 59, 64, 107, 125: all © Shutterstock

Printed and bound by in China by Toppan Leefung Printing Ltd.

Penguin Random House is committed to a sustainable future for our business,
our readers and our planet. This book is made from Forest Stewardship Council®
certified paper.

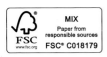